The BioChemical Machine2

The
BioChemical Machine 2

Empowering Your Body Chemistry

Eleonora De Lennart

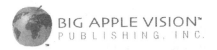

BIG APPLE VISION BOOKS
An Imprint of Big Apple Vision Publishers

The information in this book is based on the latest scientific research. However, the author and publisher are not prescribing and assume no responsibility. However, in no way should this information be considered a substitute for competent health care by the professional of your choice. In the event you use this information without your doctor's approval, you are prescribing for yourself, which is your constitutional right.

BIG APPLE VISION BOOKS
An Imprint of Big Apple Vision Publishers, New York

Library of Congress Cataloging-in-Publication Data

Copyright © 1996, 1999, 2000, 2003 by Eleonora De Lennart
ISBN: 0-9724327-8-7
www.bigapplevision.com

Fourth printing: August 2005

Big Apple Vision® is a registered trademark of Big Apple Vision Publishing, Inc.

Printed in Canada

Cover designed by George Foster
www.fostercovers.com

ACKNOWLEDGMENTS

Without courageous scientists like Professor Luke Burke, Professor Claus Leitzmann, Professor Julian Jaynes, Professor Helmut Minne, Professor Joachim Seidl, Dr. Ernest Obie, Sharon Y. Robinson, Beatrice Ymiama, M.D., James C. Romano, M.D.; inspirations like Rochelle Riservato, Michael and Moira Wehr; Herb Trimpe and Linda Fite; certified research associates like Helen Robinson; attorneys like Rebecca Millouras Lettre, and family like my husband (who shares my belief in the importance of fighting for the future of humankind), my great mother (who taught me how to fight), and the greatest sister in the world—a book like The BioChemical Machine *wouldn't have come to life.*

A very special thanks to Professor Dr. Claus Leitzmann for his involvement and guidelines for this research and to share his know-how with me for humanity.

A very special thanks to Steven LeConte Kelley, CEO and President of the Ellenville Regional Hospital, New York. He is a man with vision, who loves his country and its fellow Americans—he is also a man who turns his conviction into reality.

A very special thanks to Dr. Richard H. Dal Col, M.D.— heart surgeon extraordinaire at St. Peter's Hospital in Albany, New York.

Contents

Foreword

*By Professor Dr. Claus Leitzmann, Recipient of the Zabel
Prize for Cancer Prevention and the Broerman Prize for
Preventative Nutrition; Microbiologist, Molecular Biology
Institute, University of California; Professor, Justus Liebig
University, Giessen; Dozent in the Department of
Biochemistry and Nutrition, Mahido University, Bangkok;
(UCLA), Biochemist, author of 500 studies, articles and
books in the field of Nutrition Science*

Nobody will argue with the fact that nutrition is the
most basic requirement for our body and that the way
we eat and drink determines our health and well-being.
The question as to the most appropriate nutrition for
human has a surprisingly simple answer: Our body and
its various functions were molded by the respective
environment and by the available foods during our long
evolution. To survive, our ancestors had to be very
opportunistic and consumed any edible foodstuff that
was available that would support life and reproduction.

Modern man, living in an industrialized society
with very little physical activity, still has to be
opportunistic and select food items that will support
optimal health and well-being. Again the question about
appropriate nutrition has an astonishing straightforward
answer: Our body and its diverse functions are best
served by nutrient-dense high quality foods that have
been processed since food processing can remove or
destroy a substantial amount of the nutrients and health
promoting substances.

In practical terms this means that it is wise to prefer butter and cold-pressed plant oils rather than margarines; that it is sensible to eat egg yolk rather than egg white (sulfur-containing bad protein); and that it is prudent to consume cheese with a natural fat content rather than fat-reduced varieties, that are not only reduced in fat, but also in fat-soluble vitamins and taste.

It goes without saying that even the highest quality foods, if eaten in excess, will lead to overweight. Moderation is the simple guide that does not forego enjoyment and pleasure of eating and drinking. Another orientation that helps is to spend as much time in physical activity or outdoors as is spent watching television.

These and other valuable suggestions are part of the A&B approach and explain its overwhelming success.

Do not be led astray by emotional, commercial or political arguments, these do not help your body. *Be bold:* try it; benefit from it like other courageous people have done; propagate it to adventurous peers.

Professor Dr. Claus Leitzmann

ELLENVILLE REGIONAL HOSPITAL

Ellenville Regional Hospital
Route 209 • PO Box 668
Ellenville, NY 12428
Tel. 845-647-6400
Fax 845-647-6450

• *Member Westchester Medical Center System*

I have become a believer in the A&B method to nutrition because of personal experience and through qualitative clinical trials. I was introduced to Ms. DeLennart while she was visiting a patient at the hospital where I work. I was intrigued by the nutritional concepts and eventually was introduced to the Bio Chemical Machine book. The approach was very different than the Johnny come-lately diet fads that so many people fall for; rather the premise is based on common sense, clinical research, and historical perspective.

My administrative staff and several nurses, joined me in a qualitative study at the Ellenville Regional Hospital. What we discovered was that most individuals had small reductions in weight, had more energy, and had fewer digestion problems. We are in the process of designing more quantitative protocols to better evaluate empirical results. However, since everyone who stuck with the program feels better and does not want to stop, we will be recruiting a new set of subjects for our study. I believe the program to be so successful that we are considering offering a copy of the book and a dietary option for our hospital patients.

I was so impressed at the simplicity and efficacy of the A&B method of nutrition that I introduced it to my 74-year-old father. After reading the book and making some dietary adjustments, he has been able to completely stop using acid blocking medications for his gastro-esophageal reflux disease.

I strongly recommend the Bio Chemical Machine to everyone and keep copies in my office to share with visitors. The A&B method is easy to follow with almost no restrictions of what you may eat. You will feel better in a very short time.

Steven LeConte Kelley, CHE
President and Chief Executive Officer
Ellenville Regional Hospital

Foreword

By Dr. Quazi Al Tariq, M. D., Horton Hospital (affiliate of New York Presbyterian Hospital); Arden Hill Hospital; Mid-Hudson Forensic Psych. Center; Goshen Residential Center

"In yourself has to burn, what you want to light in other people" (Augustinus). This sentence came into my mind when I spoke to Eleonora De Lennart and read her scientifically sound research. Though the content of the book is scientific, it is entertaining, thrilling, and understandable for every layperson. I am impressed by De Lennart's findings and further development of a significant research.

In this book you will learn and understand the truth about dangerous diets, the importance of fat, the truth about cholesterol, and how to eat your food chemically perfect the easy way. It is a well-known myth that fat is bad for health. However, while reading this book, you will be surprised to learn the harsh truth about fat—that it is an integral part of our body. Without it, life is impossible. This is backed by numerous scientific researches.

It's all about chemical imbalances within the body. These imbalances lead to multiple health problems including heart disease, cancer, hyperlipidemia, and most notable, obesity. However, by eating according to the perfect match of food chemistry and body chemistry you will get total control over your health and its side effect: weight problems. By showing the history of our eating habits, De Lennart makes the logic of the research very clear. The BioChemical A&B Method® is a scientific way of eating that embraces all types of food from the rich offering of our modern world.

The BioChemical Machine is truly a comprehensive, easy to read guide for the whole family. This book is recommended for both the general reader and professionals. It is for healthy people who care for prevention and for sick people. Those who are ill will have a realistic chance to "repair" their BioChemical Machine in order to be able to look forward to a longer and happier life without pain.

It is a wonderful resource for healthy meal planning. It tackles most of the nutritional issues that concern Americans today. No matter what your age, you will find it useful and easy to understand. Beliefs about eating are changing. The focus has moved from dieting and losing weight to establishing healthful overall eating habits to help one feel good, live healthy, and prevent disease.

This book focuses on all areas of one's concern—diet, nutrition and diseases. The research is scientifically sound. This is a must-read book for every household.

Quazi Al Tariq, M.D.

GRATEFUL FOLLOWERS SAY:

"My husband went on the A&B Method® in April. So far, I have lost 22 pounds and my husband lost 26. The best part is that we both feel great..."

-Susanne B.

"I FEEL better...I'm more energetic! I love knowing about this way of eating..."

-Donna v. N.

"It's great that you care for people..."

-Muriel C.
State College PA

"I just started reading your book and I can't put it down! For about a week now I have been following the A&B Method®. I do have more energy and that is making me even more interested. I am a Physical Education teacher and I am surrounded by overweight children...! Thank you for the book and all the knowledge.

-Laura O.

"While following your program, I discovered that I was no longer lactose intolerant and my entire body experienced a renewed feeling of energy...I feel really great for the first time in many years. I also realized that I no longer have the usual menopausal symptoms, such as hot flashes, insomnia, occasional moodiness, and pains in my bones..."

-Marianne T. J.

"...It is the best I have felt in at least 10 years...My husband has severe osteoarthritis in his left knee and is eating apples and milk every day. Believe it or not, he can bend his knee now..."

-Carol. Fl.

"I love your book..."

-Susan A. L.

"…I am now just starting to eat the apples and milk again and already within a week my hip pain is almost gone…"

-Bambi T.

"…I love your book. My husband and I have been following the A&B Method®, level 2, for about two and a half weeks now. We are amazed at how much better we feel since being on it. Our energy levels have soared and our chronic muscle and joint pain have lessened tremendously. My husband has stopped napping after work every day. If we don't get our apples & milk for breakfast we crave them all day. Thank you, thank you for writing this book!! It has changed our lives already."

-Kathy R.

"…I love the milk and apple breakfast! It helped me to get rid of a strange pain…."

-Brittin C.

"…..thank you so much for writing such an informative book."

-Terry N.

"….my husband has had his transplanted kidney for 18 years. M.'s reading was once again 1.1—this is an incredible reading for a transplant patient. His doctor said it is "very rare" to have a transplanted kidney do so well [when it isn't a perfect match]. M.'s kidney was not a perfect match…M.'s creatine level was never that low until we started eating correctly following the A&B Method®. Now with two 1.1 readings in a row (six months apart), I have no doubt it is the result of the BioChemical A&B Method®..."

-Pauline C.

"…my husband and I have been following the A&B Charts® religiously and we have been symptom-free of ALL directed to the discovery of this incredible book…The chart ought to earn the author a Nobel Prize."

-K. W.

Introduction

THE CRUX OF LOSING WEIGHT: FROM "YO-YO" EFFECT TO EXHAUSTING DIETS—
Why there will NEVER be ANY Diet with a Lasting Solution (even if some of them "work"—temporarily...)

Losing weight is hard to do! Thus, dieting made losing weight big business. Yet, despite all the diet pills, slimming drinks, diet products, and never-ending guru inventions, obesity in America has reached epidemic proportions. Warnings by nutritionists and other health experts revealing the pointlessness of serial dieting have had little impact. Millions of dieters continue to torture themselves; and in the end for nothing because diets don't work. More than 95% of dieters gain all the weight back.

But the problem is in reality much bigger than just gaining back weight—not solely because most people regain even more weight than they had before—but

1

more importantly because chronic dieting weakens the immune system. It shows clearly that dieting (voluntary starvation) is not just "celebrity gossip," but a very serious matter. Something we should have to undertake once—IF at all—in a lifetime.

As I said, dieting is an unnatural state of body and mind. You are under constant stress and your Bio-Chemical Machine is unnecessarily strained as it works to prevent you from starving to death. And even if you say, "even knowing this, I will go through hell one more time, after which, I will do everything in my power to ensure that I will never gain the weight back." **The truth is: there *never has been* an effective diet; there is not an effective diet presently; but above all, there will *never be* a diet capable of providing you with a lasting solution.** You will see from the following simple, but significant reason why not even the strongest willed person can keep such a promise for longer than a couple of months let alone a year or more. Allow me to explain.

Immediately after starting a diet, the body begins decomposing: first the glycogen reserves (that are stored as blood sugar in the muscles and liver) and then the proteins. Approximately thirty hours afterwards, the glycogen is consumed. Now, the body turns to protein substances: "Glycogen from the muscles and amino acids (from which proteins are made) are being more quickly converted into blood sugar than fat reserves. At this point, you might temporarily feel a bit more "light-weighted"—but your body is definitely not as healthy as it was prior to starting a diet," explains Professor Claus Leitzmann. "This metabolic process is called ketoblastic gluconeogenesis, a process that transforms the glycogen stored in muscles into blood sugar, in relation 2:1."

> *During the first 10 days of dieting, weight reduction comes primarily from the loss of lean muscle tissue, water and glycogen—not fat as the diet industry would have you believe. Fat is the body's "ultimate reserve," tapped into only when there is nothing left for it to burn. This is the "dirty little secret" behind the success of the quick-loss fad diet doctors, their ghostwriters, and other diet gurus. In fact, the very act of dieting forces the body to "protect" its fat reserves!*

This is a protection mechanism from Mother Nature—but certainly not the mechanism you want in today's reality. *Right?* This protection mechanism is the body's natural reaction to starvation and it has been part of our BioChemical Machine for centuries. Yet, this protection mechanism also shows you the correct way out: do it slowly, but surely. Don't listen to empty promises or be fooled into believing in the latest diet craze. Medical doctors have been lending their names to programs for over 50 years and obesity still plagues America. Give your BioChemical Machine a break—a chance. Work *with*...NOT *against* Mother Nature. Successful long-term weight loss can only be achieved in cooperation with our BioChemical Machine NOT by depriving it of the food it needs.

Dieting is the voluntary act of starving and poisoning yourself. Mother Nature programmed us to WANT as much food as possible to enable us to create reserves for the bad days. But dieting runs contrary to that very basic instinct. That's what our BioChemical Machine understands. And that's what causes the negative stress. Thus, your BioChemical Machine strives to rescue you from starving to death—your body wants to survive. That's why we experience such a high degree of stress during the weeks, perhaps even months of deprivation. Simply stated, our body doesn't understand why we are undertaking something so unnatural and illogical. Early in our development, our BioChemical Machine was far more logical—when we were hungry...we ate. When hunger was satisfied...we stopped eating. Dieting is illogical. It creates bio-chemical imbalances in the body. These imbalances lead to cravings*—a reaction the body developed over eons to help prevent starvation and ensure survival. Create a perfect match between food chemistry and body chemistry and these cravings become a thing of the past!

---

* Unfortunately and despite our technological revolution, we were not able to reprogram our brain during the last 50 to 60 years when the "refrigerator- and food revolution" shook our biology. Although usually extremely flexible, our brain could not create a new part that would send signals to stop our never-ending appetite, because we are programmed exactly the other way around: eat, eat, eat! **The growth hormone ghrelin functions to increase hunger through its action on hypothalamic feeding centers.** *Ghrelin was discovered as the peptide hormone that stimulates release of growth hormone from the anterior pituitary.* **Ghrelin, along with several other hormones, has significant effects on appetite and energy balance. AND it increases plasma ghrelin concentrations observed during fasting. Ghrelin also appears to suppress fat utilization in adipose tissue, which is somewhat paradoxical considering that the growth hormone has the opposite effect.** *The predominant source of ghrelin is epithelial cells in the stomach.*

That's the big secret behind the "Yo-Yo" effect. In other words, the more you diet, the harder it becomes to lose weight. Your body learns quickly and, therefore, the next time you won't take it by surprise.

Losing weight becomes increasingly more difficult as you age. The older you are, the slower your cells perform their job. This, sooner or later, makes it impossible to solve your weight problem with any of the "traditional" diets that emphasize eliminating any of the important foods (fats, proteins and carbohydrates) necessary to healthfully maintain your BioChemical Machine. In essence, at the time of your life when losing weight makes the difference between living or not; experiencing pain or not; having energy or pathological fatigue—you are confronted with the tricky, tricky "Yo-Yo" effect—and overcoming this is no piece of cake.*

Yes, the "Yo-Yo" dilemma is a reality. As I said, it is Mother Nature's "safety net." Think of the "Yo-Yo" effect as nature's way of telling you, "don't diet, don't starve, you don't need to...." And she is right, because the BioChemical A&B Method—the perfect matching of food chemistry and body chemistry—will get you out of the vicious cycle—slowly but surely. Maybe not as quickly as you would like, but be happy because this time you can be confident that you will succeed and KNOW you will never have a relapse and even if you decide to eat "incorrectly" for a couple of days, i.e., chemically incompatible...who cares? By simply returning to the A&B principles you'll be back on track within a couple of days—THAT'S the power of the BioChemical A&B Method.

---

*And if this weren't enough, the enzyme lipase (responsible for breaking down fats into fatty acids and glycerol, produced by the pancreas) requires a slightly alkaline environment—which is not possible if you are dieting.

I am constantly receiving emails from people comparing their weight loss to others. For example, "My husband lost 26 pounds, I lost nothing." When I asked whether her husband had dieted before, the answer was "no." Others wrote, "I feel so great, but lost only one pound." I explain to people over and over again that the A&B works in phases. You may not see immediate movement on the scale, but you can be confident that your body is balancing and adjusting step-by-step. You will know this is happening because you feel a sense of renewed energy.

When it comes to those last five pounds, it might seem like your body is operating in slow motion compared to others, but that is normal. And yet, whether you are recovering from an illness or you are simply frustrated, due to a lack of results from one of those fad diets, please understand…the perfect match of food chemistry and body chemistry is the ONLY SURE way out of the "Yo-Yo" dilemma.

Glycemic Index

A couple of years ago, the famous British-born Canadian physician David Jenkins came up with the idea of creating the glycemic index for helping diabetics to choose foods that would limit the rise of their blood-sugar level. Yet, elevated blood sugar levels are your BioChemical Machine's natural reaction to food—any food. Unfortunately, Jenkins also believed (actually still believes) that the biochemical reaction to food also impacts the way the body digests food, thus influencing weight gain. But this is not the case. If the insulin does not react, just as I have described, it would mean we are nothing more than talking corpses.

The rise of your blood sugar level, especially after eating the most important energy-suppliers; (carbohydrates and fats) means your BioChemical Machine is alive and kicking. Your machine is working! Some foods elevate the sugar level more than others. This is natural in healthy people. After eating, the blood sugar level rises for a period of time and then lowers as insulin does its job. In other words, insulin* is secreted in response to rising blood sugar levels after a meal and transports sugar into the muscle cells as an energy source. That's a totally normal procedure—in healthy people.

But it's different with ill people. If their Bio-Chemical Machine is already so damaged that it cannot produce enough insulin to lower the blood sugar level, it maintains a high blood sugar level—as if something in the Machine is "stuck." In reality it is. But you cannot heal your damaged machine by just focusing on a, too often, artificially created low blood sugar level. Simply lowering the blood sugar level by avoiding exactly the food your body vitally needs to get back "on track" won't eliminate the *cause* of this problem; namely that the BioChemical Machine is in need of more serious repair. This type of repair can only be accomplished through the body's cells. And body cells are spoiled... they want something specific to eat; something they consider: "old history" food items.

That's why the theory of David Jenkins, unfortunately, helps only money hungry gurus and their

---

*Insulin is a protein hormone, produced by specialized cells in the Islets of Langerhans in the pancreas that regulate the metabolism (rate of activity) of glucose, fats, and proteins. Insulin was discovered by Frederick Banting (in 1921; another Canadian physician; Nobel Prize 1923), who pioneered its use in treating diabetes.

cash flow—not diabetics. Artificially, keeping the blood sugar level low does not mean that the BioChemical Machine is healed. Quite the contrary. Behind this "keeping it low" philosophy (and mostly eating a lot of bad proteins, see Chapter 2) the illnesses are still raging and progressing.

Being diabetic simply means: your machine is damaged—it either needs new "spare parts" or the damaged organs must be "repaired." This will be an important discussion in my next book that will be written in cooperation with one of my supporting M.D.s and the lead doctor in the BioChemical A&B Method research project at Ellenville Regional Hospital in New York.

Unfortunately, people love counting. Whatever it is: first calories and now the glycemic index of food products. Perhaps this is a result of desperation, frustration or hope that finally something will really work for the rest of their lives. In fact, this number is simply an indication of how well your body is operating at the particular point you take the reading. If your blood sugar level is low in the morning (from an empty stomach) it means your BioChemical Machine is working perfectly—which does not necessarily mean that you don't have weight problems. So what are you counting? Think about it….

Be that as it may, those who "picked up" this idea to create another, in a long line of superfluous diets, want you to believe—based on dubious studies—that this method will help you "minimize your cravings"*—

---

*Glycemic Index guru slogan

8

and provide you with the workable solution that you have been searching for. But the truth is…this is just *not* the case. It would be like saying "abracadabra" and producing medical recommendations without having the proof to back it up. To give such advice, you need the science behind the perfect match of food chemistry and body chemistry: the BioChemical A&B Charts, which I developed along with an international team of food scientists, biochemists and nutritionists.

"Healthy carbohydrates are better than unhealthy carbohydrates" is one of the oldest stories told. The reason why the glycemic index, according to some studies, "can lead to weight loss," is certainly not because some food items "release sugar slowly," but, in truth, because healthy grain, potatoes, honey and other healthy carbohydrates are the right choices for your BioChemical Machine.

At this point I would like to mention that it seems some of the diet gurus have read the European edition of my book—Copyright ©1996, and must have found my research very inspiring. Besides "borrowing" from my original concepts they sold you a package that included my well documented concepts of the "good" and "bad" carbohydrates and "good" and "bad" fats…but neglected to mention the real problem—the *"good and bad proteins."* And, most importantly left you in the dark about the revolutionary discovery that *two different types of digestion* exists for proteins; in contrast to carbohydrates. Regardless whether healthy or unhealthy—there is only *ONE* type of digestion for carbohydrates.

That's all you need to know if you want to get rid of weight and health problems for the rest of your life.

There is *no such thing* as "good" or "bad" carbohydrates! I clearly explained in my European edition why we shouldn't even call them "bad carbohydrates"—although it was my original creation to name them this way. I explained in great detail that even if some of them are *less healthy* than others, they are **never as hazardous as bad proteins,** which are central to many of today's popular diets. The real issue is the "good and bad proteins" and protein deficiency mostly caused by low-carb/high-protein diets, which sounds paradoxical (because people believe they are eating enough proteins!), but, as the research proves, are not.

That's the knowledge that will make the difference for you and millions of people. Not running like crazy, paying for unrealistic boot camps, wasting health and quality of life on senseless miracle diets and empty promises which haven't worked for as long as weight problems exist—because they *can't*, as you will learn by the end of this book.

> *Once you know how to handle the two different protein digestions you have control over your health and weight problems—forever.*

With the BioChemical A&B Method you can eat everything from potatoes and pizza to pasta, rice, chocolate, wheat bread, bananas, beer and wine *without gaining weight* but improving health and energy! As this book will inform you…addiction to carbohydrates does not mean you lack willpower or even are supposed to feel "guilty." Carbohydrate addictions (or hunger in general, especially in the night) means: your

BioChemical Machine is, in fact, starving because you didn't eat biochemically right—regardless what you have been told. Carbohydrates are *essential* for your well-being—because carbohydrates (besides fat) are the number one and two suppliers of energy! With the BioChemical A&B Method you can still love carbohydrates, and will learn how to eat them so you will no longer feel cravings of a , so-called, "addiction".

The biochemical formula for life is very simple: Eat any carbohydrate with good proteins, but never with bad proteins as you will learn throughout the book. You can eat "Neutrals" that include good protein; 24/7. This simple but significant formula will make the difference for millions of people, and will end the health and weight-related problems in this country.

Trust me...beer is great! (just to take one example among many). All this nonsense about beer, the alleged "king of all glycemic-villains" and statements like: *"The king of all sugars, the one that increases blood sugar faster than any other, is maltose, which exists in beer. Now, you understand what's behind the beer belly: The rapid rise of blood sugar caused by guzzling this beverage stimulates a corresponding rise in insulin production, which encourage storage of fat around the midsection,"* as well as *"Cooked tomatoes (in the sauce) are a great source of lycopene, a cancer fighter. Completely eliminate pizza and pasta forever and you lose two of the most palatable ways to serve this vegetable. If you can switch from deep dish to thin crust, you've made a difference... "** are making a mockery of the scientific community.

---

* South Beach Diet, page 67 and page 50

So, let's see what the *real* experts have to say on that matter:

- The American Diabetes Association refused to enter the discussion presented by the glycemic index gurus. They stated: "Studies have proven that all carbohydrates have nearly equal impact on blood sugar." And if this is the case, they do not have ANY impact on your weight! Because it would raise the simple question: Why would they?!

- "...but due to study design, the observed benefits [referring to the glycemic index] could have come from other aspects of the subjects' diets, such as fiber or overall caloric intake and for these reasons, no major health agency or professional association references glycemic index in their dietary guidelines," says David Ludwig, M.D., PhD, director of the Optimal Weight for Life (OWL) obesity program at Children's Hospital Boston. (*The Lancet*, August 28, 2004)

The uselessness of the next type of fad diet (Low-Carb) is much easier to prove. Why? Not only because 40 years of failure speaks for itself, but because it doesn't include anything about eating carbohydrates. The high-protein diet (smartly re-named low-carb diet) preceded the "renaissance" and hype of this proven failure....

Low-Carb & High-Protein Diets
(Two Sides of the Same Coin)

Desperate times require desperate measures. The industrial revolution provided us access to many wonderful new foods. As the amount of these new foods increased, so did the average American's body-weight. The diet business started booming and ignorant ideas began to flourish. But, the high-protein idea in the 1960s was ingenious...Who wouldn't be interested in a doctor who said you could lose weight by eating fried chicken, steaks and other delicious foods of this kind? So, the high-protein diet made its way around the world—especially because there was NOTHING out there that would "work" as well as stuffing your belly with meat. (to the meat industry's pleasure)

Yet serious scientists, especially those who really know how the body works, knew all along that *something was very wrong* with the high protein approach. The attacks against the diet increased, yet the high-protein approach was somehow able to survive in spite of the fact that nothing has changed since the 1960s. But something *did* change...people were *more* obese than ever and chronic illnesses were getting out of hand. The high protein approach remained mostly in diet purgatory until some creative marketing transformed it into a more saleable image and the high-protein diet became the "dernier crie"—the "low carb craze."

Everyone knows that this approach doesn't work—not only scientists, but the diet industry as well. Yet, since so many people confused the loss of muscle and water with success, they truly believed the program worked for over 40 years.

Atkins, for example, based his credo on the following theory: "Atkins develops the hypothesis that the diet he proposes is the diet that humans have evolved to eat." (Harvard Health letter, August 2004.) Not only is this wrong, (see Chapter 1, "The Perfect Match of Food Chemistry & Body Chemistry,") but we wouldn't be alive if our ancestors really lived this way. IF it was really this simple WHY isn't everyone in the world already slim and healthy?—Because our early ancestors didn't eat meat as portrayed, they cracked the bones in order to eat the ("NEUTRAL") marrow. Later ancestors viewed animals as walking "food producers"—and not meant to be slaughtered. Our ancestors lived healthfully from the animals products— which is why you will find them in the "24/7 NEUTRAL" section on the BioChemical A&B Charts.

And so, the serious scientific studies revealed the following:

- Followers of the [Atkins] diet suffer from muscle cramps, diarrhea, general weakness, and rashes more frequently than people on low-fat diets. (*The Lancet*, September 4, 2004)

- One year after dieting, people gain more weight back. Low-carb diets are not more effective than any other diet, says Dr. Walter Willet, Harvard School of Public Health (CNN, May 18, 2004)

- "Low-carb diets may be dangerous to your long-term health!" (*Heart Center Online*, 2004)

OK, we all know that reports on most studies end with a sentence "…more research is needed," or as it has been published in regard to the Atkins diet: "Arne Astrup and colleagues say more research is needed on the Atkins diet." (*The Lancet*, September 4, 2004) Perhaps another 40 years, an 80% national obesity rate and the bankruptcy of the Medicare system will complete the research!

Fact is that carbohydrates are vital for our well-being, energy, health AND proper weight. You can't sustain weight loss without eating healthy carbohydrates, such as wheat bread, potatoes, honey, and others. If you try, your body will try to "rescue" you—with cravings—from starving. In truth, gaining weight by eating carbohydrates is an "artificial weight gain." Within a couple of days you are back on track anyway.

Therefore, there is only one question left: Why do some people believe that fad diets work? Because they provide instant gratification and temporary weight loss—but only if you are satisfied to lose muscle mass, glycogen and water….

Why Do Some Diets Work—Temporarily?

After studying countless books from so called diet "experts," I came to realize that their hook is basically deprivation. Most gurus instruct you to omit significant food groups from your day-to-day diet. One vilifies dairy products; another, carbohydrates; and others, proteins in their entirety. Or fat, oil, saturated fat and cholesterol are the "main villain." And if it's no longer cholesterol and saturated fat, well, then they'll find another scapegoat, like casein,* to become the root of all evil.

Once they've got you hooked, fad diets sell you on the idea that you need "urgent" cleansing. But many of these detoxification programs are based primarily on a lot of bad or extremely-bad protein and almost all require giving up certain food groups. In short, they are based on a type of starvation.** Gurus "prescribe" these high protein diets—heavily promoted today as low carb diets—because it is the easiest way for them to make money.

The excessive eating of extremely-bad protein, the worst of the acid-builders, is not what your metabolism requires. Your body needs base-forming foods— alkalinity—to counteract the acid debris released into the circulation when cells die. If we eat too much protein and too little carbohydrates and fat, the body is forced to obtain its energy from protein, especially the extremely-bad protein that is only an emergency supplier to our metabolism. See Step #2 from the Big Seven Essentials. (See Part II, Chapter 5.) Eating too much extremely-bad protein drains your alkaline reserve and your BioChemical Machine suffers.

Why Do Harmful Fad Diets Persist?

People continue to buy into fad diets because of short-term results—instant gratification that comes from eliminating major food groups. But let's face it—

---

* Casein is present in milk as calcium-salt and creates the milky color. It is the main protein of milk, from which it can be separated by the action of acid, the enzyme rennin, or bacteria (souring). Milk contains amino acids and phosphoric acids. Phosphate salts or esters of phosphoric acid are involved in many biochemical processes, often as part of complex molecules.

**Acidosis is a very prominent condition in starvation. When base-forming foods are withheld from the digestive tract, there is nothing to tie or bind the acids and we get the acid build-up found in starvation.

nobody can go forever without bread, macaroni (especially macaroni and cheese), potatoes, rice, noodles, pasta and pizza. *Right?* Healthy carbohydrates (from Groups I and II, see Chapter 5) are our body's #2 energy supplier; especially after 50. More to the point...we love eating them!

Yet thirty years after I, myself, tried the dangerous high-protein diets without success. I couldn't believe what was happening: the (extremely-bad) protein diet from the 1960s was back. Why? The answer is simple, but significant: With high protein diets, you eat foods like those from the "B" column; foods like those from the "Neutral" column, but *completely eliminate carbohydrates from the "A" column.* (See Chart, Chapter 4.)

That's why unhealthy, high-protein food-combining diets work for a while—because by eating a lot of cooked meats (extremely-bad protein) you are *partially* eating according to the A&B principles—but *NOT* the *actual BioChemical A&B Way!* What this means is you are eating too many bad proteins; you are losing muscle and water—*NOT* fat; and if this isn't enough...you are poisoning yourself and opening yourself up to develop protein deficiency.

Unfortunately, once you resume your normal eating habits (incompatible eating of meat, bread, macaroni, potatoes, rice, noodles, pasta, and pizza, which is not the BioChemical A&B way) you can't keep the pounds off.

Then there's another popular diet that is the exact opposite—dictating that you should eat *only* carbohydrates with some foods from the "Neutral" column and completely eliminate proteins from your diet. *Again, you are eating, partially, according to the A&B principles;* and again, that's why it works for a short time. So with this type of diet, you can eat whole wheat bread, potatoes, couscous, brown rice, and whole wheat noodles with vegetables, salads and fruits...but you are *NOT* allowed to eat fat, vital good proteins, such as "Neutral" meat and "Neutral" fish, and whole milk and other vital dairy products. If you like milk and dairy products, according to these gurus you are "suckling a cow." There is *NO* distinction between good, bad, and extremely-bad proteins or the tremendous importance of milk to our health.

The Confusion Gurus Created by Distorting Hay's Original Research

The problem with most diet programs is that gurus have purposely dissected Dr. Hay's original research, see "In the Name of Science." They've taken a little from here and a little from there to cobble together diets that have more to do with marketing than your health. From scientifically sound research on how to maintain a proper acid-alkaline balance; they oversimplified Dr. Hay's work to invent a fashionable—and completely misleading—new concept: food combining.

Eating carbohydrates and proteins at the same time is our nature. It is not important how much protein or carbohydrate a food item contains (as Index-guru counters explain)—what *is* important is how your BioChemical Machine is able to cope with certain food items; the old history and new history food items, see Chapter 1. The BioChemical A&B Method is about dealing with *new* food items—food items that historically played no role in the development of our body's chemistry.

In the framework of the A&B principles, all food items are classified according to the perfect match with our body's chemistry and its two different types of protein digestion. You will find vegetables in three different groups; fruits in three different groups; dairy products in two different groups; meat, fish, and nuts in three different groups. Even the egg is divided in two different groups.

Diet gurus, on the other hand, classify meat, fish, eggs and dairy products in one group only: "proteins." This is wrong. Matching food chemistry with body chemistry is just not that simple! This is why these food-combining gurus omit significant food groups as a whole and don't even separate the correct food items.

The BioChemical A&B Method is NOT about separating or eliminating foods. If you follow the distorted advice of diet gurus, then you go on and on unknowingly eating incompatible food, never ridding your body of toxins, and then wonder why losing weight is so difficult. Fad diets don't work because they *do not* eliminate the cause of obesity, fatigue, and disease: self-poisoning. You can torture yourself for a few weeks following their strict regimens and being unbearably hungry, but you'll probably join the more than 95% of dieters who eventually lapse back into their old ways.

Even if you muster enough willpower to follow a strict diet regimen, the day will come when you'll find yourself unable to lose any more weight. *The laws of body chemistry upset your fad diet and then you are stuck!* And remember the "YO-YO" EFFECT: the more diets you try, the less you will be able to lose weight. You will gain everything back plus *more*. And remember…you lose only muscle mass, glycogen and water.

All fad diets are stressful, but they also trigger hazards to your health.

"Most such [fad] diets...are ineffective and sometimes much worse...and could put heart patients at risk in the long-term. Short-term success adds to the diets' allure. Some fad diets induce temporary weight loss just by restricting calories or imposing a monotony that kills the appetite. Others bring about water loss with their high-fat, low carbohydrate content.

But extreme dieting can pose dangers. The fast fat-burning caused by drastic diets releases ketones, or acids, into the blood, in a process called ketosis. Excess ketosis can damage your health and can even put dieters with diabetes into a coma."

—Marilyn Chase, "Health Journal," *The Wall Street Journal*, April 7, 1997, page B1.

Chase is right. Most fad diets require starving and starvation causes acidosis. You will not only have difficulty losing weight, because you are starving, but are also poisoning your cells, i.e., yourself.

"Ketogenic diets cause a loss of body water, sodium and potassium. Dieters can experience dizziness, or elevated uric acid putting them at risk for kidney stones and gout. At worst, an electrolyte imbalance from mineral loss can trigger heart-rhythm disturbances. We've had people [who] passed out after losing too many minerals."

—Ellen Coleman, a dietitian in Riverside, California, quoted in the "Health Journal" section of *The Wall Street Journal*, April 7, 1997.

Without knowledge of the matching food chemistry and body chemistry there is no lasting solution; regardless of what you have been promised. As we grow older the struggle to lose weight through fad diets only grows more difficult. Remember the law of our body chemistry: beginning at age thirty, cell activity begins to slow down more and more with each passing decade.

Chemically perfect eating is possible, even in our modern world, if we apply a new way of thinking about food. Following the perfect match between food chemistry and body chemistry is a way of life—not a temporary fix. *Because it is NOT about food—it is about your cells.* In the words of Kathy Quinn, Patient Care Services Coordinator at the Ellenville Hospital, New York who participated in the scientific clinical study, "I consider myself a walking cell." And she's right.

Cells are not negotiable. If we understand this, we know we don't need eating plans, diets, non-diets, anti-diets, food-combiners, glycemic indexes, low-carb, low-fat, high-protein, blood-type or whatever never-ending ideas make a lot of people rich—on your account. Because dieting is the enemy of your health and, in the final analysis, even of your perfect weight.

In the next chapter, "In the Name of Science", you will read the story about my fateful encounter with Professor Luke Burke at Rutgers University, his challenging involvement that lead to the groundbreaking discovery of the perfect match of food chemistry and body chemistry—and its two different types of protein digestion.

The BioChemical A&B Method is the perfect match of food chemistry and body chemistry. It is the result of many years of research. It is the "guide" to help people's "old" body chemistry (developed over the course of millions of years) to handle the labyrinth of today's (delicious and seductive) "modern" foods, which have been invented after World War II when refrigerators revolutionized the food industry and made "modern" food items possible.

With the BioChemical A&B Method you can eat everything and anything, including bad proteins and extremely-bad proteins that are, in fact, the cause of many health and weight problems. Yet, the BioChemical A&B Method teaches how to eat unhealthy foods so that they don't harm your BioChemical Machine.

And here is the story of my discovery that will free you from the crux of losing weight forever...

- *In the following chapters, you will see that I'll mention notions such as acid-alkaline balance and pH (potential of hydrogen) in connection to Dr. Hay's groundbreaking research about the acid-alkaline balance. Please be advised that the BioChemical A&B Method is not an "acid-alkaline diet" or "pH diet," or any of these diets— it is the perfect match of food chemistry and body chemistry.*

- *Also, the BioChemical A&B Charts are not acid-alkaline charts (as many diet gurus, who are using years of research for their useless diets, assumed). You will see alkaline-building as well as acid-building food items in all three BioChemical A&B Chart columns.*

- *Moreover, acid-building food items are divided into two different groups: unhealthy and healthy acid-builders, which produce vast differences to your digestive system.*

- *AND you will see that there is a BioChemical A&B Chart LEVEL ONE for healthy people—where the division of alkaline or acid-building foods doesn't play any role at all!*

- *The vital acid-alkaline balance is only part of this research.*

- *Again, the very foundation of the BioChemical A&B Method is built upon the groundbreaking discovery of the good and bad proteins; the two different protein digestions; **and protein deficiency, which can be avoided once you know how to eat bad proteins correctly.** It is your "guide" to handle the labyrinth of today's delicious and seductive foods. Once you know how to handle the TWO DIFFERENT PROTEIN DIGESTIONS you have control over your health and weight problems—for the rest of your life.*

23

IN THE NAME OF SCIENCE

Although he is not a clergyman, I believe Luke Burke, PhD, a professor at Rutgers University in New Jersey, will one day be seen as a saint to millions of Americans. Currently chairman of the Department of Chemistry, Dr. Burke played an instrumental role in a revolutionary discovery that I believe will provide millions of people with the necessary information for solving their most challenging health and weight problems.

Prior to my first meeting with Professor Burke, PhD, I became aware of his commanding reputation by Sharon Robinson. Robinson, a senior chemist at the New Jersey Department of Health, had come to realize that my work had the potential to help millions of people. However, before I presented him with my research that clarified and expanded on the acid-alkaline balance research of William Howard Hay for his critique, she warned me about her mentor: "Nothing unscientific! No imperfections!"

Up to this point, I had not yet made the groundbreaking discovery of the concept of the good and bad proteins, and that two different types of protein digestion exist. This, you will learn is the root of many, if not all, health and weight evils of our modern times. Like many of the "diet gurus," whose theories I scorned, I was stuck with the tired and unscientific message of "separating carbohydrates and proteins." And yes, even though I had already completed the original A&B Chart, it was still not *the* revolutionary match of food chemistry and body chemistry—the method you'll find on the BioChemical A&B Charts included in this book.

Yes, there were many moments when I deeply regretted ever having touched this project. I had no idea what I was getting myself into or what I was putting at risk.* But ultimately, I am happy that I did what I had to do because it has already positively impacted thousands of lives; including those of my husband, my sister, my mother, my mother-in-law and yes, my own. Beyond that, it made life worth living! A life without pain, ailments, fatigue, and a life where there is no daily struggle with something we all love to do—namely, eating.

My Personal Journey

Twenty years ago, I began a journey that I am convinced saved my life. In my early 20s, I was in great shape, energetic and slim. But as I grew older, I began to struggle with a variety of health problems. I was plagued by fatigue and pain caused by what I would

---

*I did it because of "the trillions of dollars for health-care costs in a world that quadrupled in population in one century…and it's heading for 9 to 10 billion." *Time*, November 1, 1999, page 87

"In the year 2021, every American will be overweight. Health care costs…will reach $16 trillion by the year 2020." American Heart Association, 9/1998.

later learn to be self-poisoning. I suffered through a litany of ailments, from liver, pancreas, and kidney diseases to diabetes, tumors, fatigue, and clinical depression. Making matters worse, I struggled with my weight and the associated frustrations of ineffective diets and useless "magic" pills.

I didn't realize that I was already caught up in the most vicious and telltale cycles of our very existence: pathological fatigue. This is the first sign that something is wrong with the balance of the body chemistry. And I certainly didn't know that the causes of fatigue are closely related to the causes of disease. As I would learn, pathological fatigue is the result of unknowingly poisoning oneself through "chemically incompatible" eating.

Furthermore, increasing weight problems, and the subsequent involvement with alleged "miracle diets," took their toll. Like many others confronted with similar health ailments, I bought into false claims that did nothing more than complicate my problems.

Finally, in the summer of 1983, I hit a low point in my life. I was experiencing pain in every fiber of my body and was so weak that I could hardly walk. It was late in the evening and I remember thinking I needed professional help and I needed it fast. But, because of the hour, I could not contact my regular physician. In retrospect, this turned out to be a blessing in disguise because it led me to call my friend John Blair M.D., a specialist in internal medicine. He was one of those incredibly dedicated professionals who attend every key seminar around the country that focuses on the latest medical research. I was hopeful he would be able to offer me something new: Perhaps a miracle pill or at least information on the latest revolutionary medical procedure or treatment.

Instead, he introduced me to a way of approaching food that would change my life forever. After examining my, formerly energetic body, he asked about my eating habits. Then, instead of prescribing the expected medication, he pulled a little book from his pocket...*A New Health Era* by William Howard Hay, M.D.[1] He explained that the cause of my fatigue and body pains could be directly attributed to an imbalance in my body chemistry and that the book outlined a method of learning to live with food in a way that would bring my body chemistry back into alignment. I was surprised, and admittedly, *very* disappointed.

Not only had I never heard of this Dr. Hay, I had no interest in trying any more diet programs.

But Blair stressed that this was *not* a diet. "It's a scientifically documented method for smart eating," he said. "It's about your body chemistry and serves as both prevention and cure...as a side effect, your weight will take care of itself."

I had heard this promise before. I couldn't imagine that something as ordinary as food could be the solution to my health and weight problems. Yet, I knew I could trust John and above all, I felt so ill, that I decided to follow his instructions even though I was sure they would fail.

Dr. William Howard Hay

Dr. William Howard Hay graduated from New York University on March 26, 1891, and practiced medicine and general surgery (see appendix). Many of his original guidelines are still employed by nutritionists and dieticians. His focus was the acid-alkaline balance and his advice was simple: eat what nature offers. In Dr. Hay's day, his approach was sound since life (and food) was still pretty simple. There were no fast food restaurants and no super size supermarkets with unimaginable numbers of delicious and mouthwatering products. Instead, we shopped at "Mom & Pop shops" like the neighborhood butcher and other small grocery markets. Smaller incomes and simpler times meant less availability of the types of foods that are so damaging to our BioChemical Machine.

Be that as it may, that very night I didn't think about bygone times; I just did as my physician suggested. I changed my eating habits and almost immediately began feeling better. It was almost like the cartoon figure Popeye, who, after eating his spinach, experiences an immediate reaction. After a few days, my energy began to return and, slowly but surely, the strange pains in my body began to lessen. I was stunned and didn't know what to make of it…but I stuck to the method religiously. I lost 25 pounds in six weeks and slowly began overcoming the other health problems that had plagued me for so long. As long as I ate properly choosing foods based on their chemical compatibility— I continued to make progress. It didn't matter if I ate baked potatoes with butter, wheat bread with mayonnaise, or pizza with olives—the program worked! *Little did I know at the time… the best was yet to come.*

As I moved into my 40s, my life was better than ever. Unfortunately, I was unaware that there was a new horror lurking around the corner that would plague my life with 24-hour pain; rheumatoid arthritis. As the illness progressed, my thumb became crippled and the pain in my bones, especially my hipbones, increased dramatically. I needed a cane to get up from the couch. Despite heavy painkillers the pain didn't stop. Finding no relief from traditional treatments I started to research the illness. I couldn't understand why this was happening to my body after eating correctly for so long.

For many years, I had avoided drinking milk because of its pesticides, chemicals, and hormones. I have no doubt that eliminating it from my diet played a big part in my body's calcium deficiency.

However, the more I researched, the more I realized this was not the whole cause of my affliction. If it was, all arthritic and osteoarthritic cases could be cured by drinking more milk and eating more dairy products. Unfortunately it's not that simple.

In retrospect, it was the key experience of researching my rheumatoid arthritis (or rather my panic over seeing my crippled thumb and imagining this happening to the rest of my body) that led to my most important and landmark discovery—the vast chemical differences between *"good"* and *"bad" proteins* and the discovery that two different types of digestion exists for protein—one for the *good proteins* (pure/high grade protein) that the human body has evolved to handle over the course of millions of years; another for *bad proteins* (abnormal proteins), which have been consumed in larger and larger quantities only since the invention of home refrigeration; and their impact on the health of our BioChemical Machine.

Knowing the distinction between these proteins and understanding how to counteract their impact on your overall health and weight will empower you to control your body's vitality.

Having experienced the positive impact of Hay's work, I wondered why everyone didn't know about it.

When I looked closer, I found the answer. As a result of his research on the acid-alkaline balance and alkaline reserve, Hay had concluded that the root of all physical (and psychological) evil is directly related to the body's chemical imbalance. "All forms of disease and weight problems fall under one heading—chemical imbalance."[2]

Such revolutionary investigations and discoveries have been known to lead to a Nobel Prize. But that wasn't the case here. On the contrary, the scientific community dismissed his groundbreaking research!

As I would soon discover, there was an obstacle that allowed the quacks to distort Hay's work. Although his revolutionary research was primarily about acid-alkaline balance, he simplified part of the food chemistry findings and spoke of "separating carbohydrates from proteins."

This was his biggest mistake. Simply put, it was unscientific. Almost every food item consists of proteins and carbohydrates at the same time. Yet, even if his conclusions were partially wrong, his basic premise was still sound. For the scientific community, however, results must be perfect, which was not the case with Dr. Hay's findings.

Therefore, until recently we had missed out on the benefits of his research. I truly believe Hay's findings were largely responsible for saving my life. I also believe that the combination of Hay's work and my expansion of his basic research can benefit millions of people, not only in terms of prevention, but also to escape the vicious cycle of gurus and their never-ending miracle diets. I am living proof of the program's success, as are so many others. Everyone I convinced to try the BioChemical A&B Method has succeeded. Ultimately, it was the program's simple success, and not the need for scientific proof, that served as my driving force.

However, I knew it was proof that would ultimately return Hay's reputation to good standing in the scientific community.

Dr. Hay didn't involve food chemists in his work, as he should have, and he oversimplified terms to enable ordinary people to profit from his research. That was good thinking, but, *and here is the big **but**...*at the same time he created a loophole for those who would make billions of dollars by shamelessly using only portions (especially the wrong ones!) of his findings. Gurus shaped his research into hazardous, ill-advised diets. Forty years after his death, Hay was dismissed as a quack. He became the father of all food-combining gurus, diet *du jour* starlets, and nutritionist wannabes. Whoever speaks of "food-combining diets" or "combination diets" or urges you to omit certain food groups has distorted Dr. Hay's beneficial research. Unwittingly, despite his good intentions, Dr. Hay—the originator of scientific eating—had inspired money-hungry people to turn the BioChemical Machine into a money making machine.

Dr. Hay's findings about the acid-alkaline balance and the vital alkaline reserve should be considered a major research finding. Unfortunately, Dr. Hay had come up with the right idea at the wrong time; a time when the pharmaceutical industry was on the rise and the focus was on cure, not prevention or side effects. Propaganda hammered miracle drugs into our parents' minds until they and the following generations believed that a pill could do anything. But we know this is just not true. My desire to clarify the misconceptions about Dr. Hay's research—and bring his findings to light—

32

grew into a driving passion. Above all, I wanted to clear his reputation within the scientific community.

And so, with a lot of conviction and after a lot of hard work (that included developing the BioChemical A&B Chart by conferring with an international team of food scientists, biochemists and nutritionists), I did what I had to do as the first step to restoring Dr. Hay's good name: I reached out to the scientific community. As I said, Sharon Robinson of the New Jersey Department of Health, introduced me to Luke Burke, Professor of Biochemistry, and warned me of his intractability when it came to scientific facts. But, since I was about to resurrect seriously significant research, I decided that Professor Burke was the right person to contact.

In the summer of 1997, I called Professor Burke, sent him my work, and arranged an appointment. When I entered his modern office for the first time, he was very kind; no question about it. He was much taller, younger, and sportier than I'd anticipated, but precisely as sharp as one would expect of such a highly respected scientist. I felt that he didn't *really* know what to think of me. Here I was, full of passion to help humankind; anxiously awaiting his reaction to my work. On top of his desk sat my open manuscript. He looked at the book as if to confirm he had received something so unscientific from me. After all, high-profile professors from Princeton University, Munich University, New Jersey State College, Denver University, and Hagia Academy had, previously, endorsed my other major research documented in my book, *The Race That Should Be Human*.

"Do you *really* believe that separating carbohydrates from proteins is the solution for health and weight problems? That's nonsense! I can't associate my name with something unscientific like that," he thundered.

Obviously, he had already made up his mind. I knew that if I couldn't convince this hard-evidence-oriented scientist, Dr. Hay's research would always remain in the dim zone of quacks. I told Professor Burke that I truly believed I would be dead if I had not discovered and followed this program over the past 15 years. I related my litany of surgeries and the agony of trying every diet from high-protein to pills. I presented him with test results gathered by the German physician, Dr. Ludwig Walb, one of the doctors who attempted to prove Dr. Hay's research correct. These publications didn't impress him at all.

"If this were serious research," Professor Burke said, "I would have received it directly from the scientists or the institutions themselves. That's the usual procedure." To demonstrate, he showed me a letter about other medical research sent by German researchers, which he had received that very same day, as well as some papers from the Max Planck Institute in Germany.

"But perhaps they didn't understand how it works?" I said, trying to defend Dr. Walb's good intentions to spread Dr. Hay's teachings. I sensed an invisible wall surrounded Professor Burke, separating him from my passion. I realized that I was defending myself while fighting for the truth of something that I wholeheartedly believed in. I realized that it was most likely the endorsement of Professor Julian Jaynes of Princeton University or the book's title that explained why Professor Burke decided to meet with me in the first place. I know the title of the book had caught his attention. He liked my idea of comparing the body to a

BioChemical Machine very much. Despite his skepticism, there was something about my work that held his attention.

All of a sudden, he interrupted my thoughts and asked: "Why are you doing this project?"

"Because I'm so angry," I said and pointed to his computer, which in a moment of frustration, I confused with a television. I explained to him that the misleading ads on TV were making me angry, but I was especially angry with medical doctors who used their image to sell dangerous diets in order to make millions of dollars, often without regard for people's lives.* "More than 100,000 Americans will die this year alone due to improper eating habits,"[3] I said. "Most people don't understand that heartburn is the first sign of chronic disease in the making. They don't realize that fatigue, illness, and obesity are all intertwined. Americans are increasingly overweight, and we must do something about escalating health-care costs. It's as important as solving our environmental problems. It's as important as solving our political problems. It's about future generations. It's about changing minds, and it's also about health consciousness."

I went on to tell him about my research and my conviction to contribute whatever I could to help solve the problems of this dramatically changing world in this new millennium. "Everyone who learns to balance his or her own body chemistry will profit from it and will have the same energy as I have today," I explained.

"How can you prove what you say?" he said.

"I am the living proof!" I replied.

"But that's not scientific," he said, smashing my explanations. Gotcha!

35

And so, with all my remaining energy, I tried one more time to convince the man whom I hoped would help me get this research into the right hands at American universities, and ultimately, the scientific community. "I found a cure for arthritis!" I suddenly said. "I developed a milk and apple therapy, a natural miracle drug!" And I added, "You probably don't know what it means to be in pain day in and day out." I was determined that I wouldn't leave his office until I had convinced him to introduce me to other scientists. This was my goal.

I told him about people who had benefited from the BioChemical A&B Method, people who at one time could not walk or live without painkillers. I spoke of my mother-in-law, who had been scheduled for surgery, but canceled the procedure due to her remarkable recovery; and I told him about my dentist's husband, who was scheduled for hip surgery and, after two weeks of following the A&B Method, came dancing to my house.

"They have medical records in black and white!" I told Professor Burke. "I myself needed a cane to get up from a chair before I began this method of eating." Burke looked at me, trying to figure out whether I was telling the truth, since I walk like a young girl.

"This program works. I know that the theory of separating carbohydrates from proteins is an over-simplification of great research, but I also know there is something here," I told Professor Burke.

He looked into my eyes and said, "Well, then, go and find it and then come back."

---

*Those who promote diet products, slimming drinks and diet pills contribute to a $32 billion dollar industry.

53% suffer from chronic pain. ABC World News, May 8, 2005

225,000 die each year in America of cardiac arrest. ABC May 3, 2005.

36

During the following weeks, I worked feverishly polishing my research. When I walked with my beloved German Shepherd, Quinky, I had only one question on my mind: what is behind the theory of separating proteins from carbohydrates? It was during a follow-up meeting with Professor Burke that he came up with something I had not immediately recognized as revolutionary.

"The A&B principles are very interesting," he said, referring to my A&B Chart. "You don't separate the proteins from the carbohydrates."

I looked at him, speechless. This was the missing link!

On my return trip home, my mind was completely occupied with Professor Burke's words. Once home, I stormed into my office, ignoring the joyful greetings of my dog, to review the A&B Chart. Burke was right! On the chart, I had not separated carbohydrates from proteins. According to their chemistry, I had put vegetables into three groups, fruits in three, meat in two, fish in two, dairy products in two, nuts in two, and even eggs into two groups. Carbohydrates themselves were divided into three groups. In addition, I had an additional group, the "Neutrals", which included selected dairy, meat, and fish products that, according to most diet gurus, should not be eaten with carbohydrates, vegetables, fruits, and nuts.

This was it! By trial and error I had discovered sound scientific principles to support the BioChemical A&B Method. This perfect match of food chemistry and body chemistry maintains the vital alkaline buffer that supports the proper balance of acid and alkalinity in the blood, which in turn prevents us from poisoning ourselves. At that moment, it became clear to me that this omission was the primary reason Dr. Hay never received his Nobel Prize. Now, instead of looking solely toward genetic engineering and other expensive interference with our BioChemical Machine, we can employ the simplest and most satisfying thing in the world—food—to dramatically improve our health.

Initially, it was Professor Burke's intractability that challenged me to further develop Dr. Hay's findings. Soon after, my completed research was to receive support from eminent authorities such as Professor Helmut Minne (A), Professor Claus Leitzmann (B), Steven LeConte Kelley (C), Dr. Quazi Al-Tariq (D), Dr. Beatrice Inyama (D), and Dr. Ernest Obie (D). These respected members of the scientific and medical establishment had originally refused to endorse Dr. Hay's research. Professor Helmut Minne had even called it "hocus-pocus." Today, Professor Helmut Minne and others enthusiastically endorse and support my work.

Patients of other physicians (E) have benefited from the A&B Method to alleviate the effects of such conditions like diabetes, obesity, heart disease, cancer, kidney disease, arteriosclerosis, arthritis, osteoporosis, rheumatism, allergies, thyroid and cholesterol problems, ulcers, even multiple sclerosis (in combination with electro-neural-therapy, acc. to Croon (F).)

Now—so can you!

Yet, before you will begin one of the most important journeys of your life—a voyage that will change your and your family's life forever, let me discuss one of the saddest chapters in the history of humankind…A chapter that must be "closed" as soon as possible: *Obesity in Children.* I received tons of wonderful emails from people who told me how much their entire family loves the A&B Method—including their children. Some wrote that they couldn't imagine how they ever lived without eating "Milk & Apples" in the morning (containing the same amount of fiber as a whole bowl of cereal!); that their children would learn so much easier at school (and wouldn't fall asleep) and that energy and joy had entered their homes.

The BioChemical A&B Method is, in fact, a family affair. Many men also wrote me and women who told me "that their husband was even *more* into it," and, as I said, their children loved it—*Why*? Because they can eat anything they want; just the BioChemical A&B way.

(A) Professor Helmut Minne, M.D., University of Heidelberg, Chairman of the Board of Directors of the Kuratorium Knochengesundheit [bone health], e.V./Clinic Der Fuerstenhof, Bad Pyrmont.
(B) Professor Claus Leitzmann, Zabel Prize for Cancer Prevention; Broermann Prize for Preventative Nutrition; Molecular Biology Institute, University of California; Microbiology and BioChemistry, University of Minnesota; Dozent in the Department of Biochemistry and Nutrition, Mahido University, Bangkok; Director of the Research Laboratory of Anemia and Malnutrition Research Center, Chaing Mai, Thailand; Professor of Nutrition, Justus Liebig University; author of about 500 publications and books in the field of Nutrition Science. Among them, the "Dictionary of Nutrition," translated into English, French, Italian and Spanish (Ulmer).
(C) Steven LeConte Kelley, research scientist at Rensselaer Polytechnic Institute and Albany Medical Center, New York; CEO and President of the Ellenville Hospital, New York.
(D) Dr. Quazi Al-Tariq, M.D., Horton Hospital (affiliate of New York Presbyterian), Arden Hill Hospital, Mid Hudson Forensic Psyc. Center, Goshen Residential Center. (D) Dr. Beatrice Inyama, M.D., Toledo Hospital. (D) Ernest Obic, M.D., Medical Expert/ Consultant to the United Nations.
(E) Dr. Ragnar Berg,[4] the chemist, Fred W. Koch, Dr. Friedrich Sander,[5] Professor Louis-Claude Vincent, Dr. Berthold Kern, Dr. Michael Worlitschek, Dr. Eduard A. Brecht[6] Dr. Hermann Aihara,[7] Professor Lothar Wendt, Dr. Bircher-Brenner,[8] Professor W. Zabel, Dr. Ludwig Walb.
(F) Physicians Journals for Nature Cure, 38-9/1997. In combination with electro-neural-therapy and several methods of holistic therapy.

The BioChemical A&B Method will *not* interfere with **MEDICAL TREATMENTS**. On the contrary, this program is designed to **ENHANCE** its **EFFECTIVENESS**.

As with any new program, first consult with your physician before starting the BioChemical A&B Method.

OBESITY IN CHILDREN

"*O*besity *in children and adolescents is a serious issue with many health and social consequences... which continue into adulthood,*" stated The American Obesity Association. Children are the last people in this world who should need diets! Why? Because children's cells are supposed to work properly and at full potential. Additionally, their physical activity usually equals their food intake. Sadly, the reality of 2005 is different. Childhood obesity has reached epidemic proportions. Diabetes in children and other illnesses have become so common that most people believe that this isn't unusual, but "normal." However, having diabetes means simply, your BioChemical Machine is damaged, which is almost unimaginable at a young age—when cells are supposed to be at their most optimum level.

Worst of all, children are even ready to staple their stomachs in order to be "like the others" who have no weight problems. Nobody can really predict what the consequences of stomach stapling will be in years to come—regardless of what some physicians say. Not only is there long-term research data available, but it doesn't take a fortune-teller (but honest researchers, who are supposed to be one step ahead of physicians) to

"predict" what might happen in 20, 30, 40 or 50 years—
if there will *be* 50 years ahead of these people who were
driven by desperation to take the road of such drastic
measures.

I can't repeat often enough—that the heart of the
matter and biggest problem of our time is NOT about
FOOD—it IS about CELLS. Our problem is not "guilt,"
lack of willpower, and all these nonsensical excuses—it
is about learning and following the laws of our body
chemistry. It is about the fact that our body digests good
protein differently than bad proteins. *This is the
breakthrough discovery.* Knowing this, you can rule
your body—AND the body of your child. No boot
camp, no low-carb, no low-fat, no-low-whatsoever can
help you in the long run—NOR does it help your child!
You are the parent; *you* have the power to help your
child learn to eat properly from childhood so their adult
lives will be healthy.

You can't stop your child from wanting to go into
fast food restaurants, enjoying their McWho-ever-it-is,
milk shakes, French fries, apple pies and chocolate. But
you *can* teach your child how to eat them right! And
here is the catch that will make the difference: If your
child's cells receive the right foundation (for the cells)
AT HOME, it will strengthen the immune system and
even eating fast food from time to time will not be able
to cause lasting damage in your child's BioChemical
Machine.

Also, if your child would eat according to the
requirements of his or her body chemistry, s/he will not
develop carbohydrate addiction and certainly won't
suffer from cravings for certain foods, which is usually
connected to carbohydrate addiction from chemical
imbalance.

As previously stated, I received many, many emails from parents who told me how much their children loved the Milk & Apple breakfast, that they would no longer be tired after breakfast; and that their learning problems had dramatically improved. They also reported that their children did not even realize that they are eating chemically right; they just loved it!

Nobody could live according to a diet plan forever—but there is certainly no child in this world who could or would want to do it. Just be a role model for your child and your family about how much joy eating can bring, so that the perfect match of food chemistry and body chemistry will become "normal" for future generations. If you do this—you will liberate your child from what our generation went through—needing "gurus" to feed our cells in order to exist...

PART I

THE HISTORY OF THE PROBLEM

Good, Bad, and Extremely-Bad
Proteins—The *Real* Story

Chapter 1

THE PERFECT MATCH BETWEEN FOOD CHEMISTRY & BODY CHEMISTRY
The History of Good Proteins and the Birth of Bad and Extremely-Bad Proteins

It is no secret that we human beings have clear-cut rules about our biology and chemistry. And, of course, we all know that we are part of the zoological class Mammalia, which evolved from mammal-like reptiles roughly 200 million years ago.[9]

But what you may not know, and a crucial point to remember is this: as mammals, our body chemistry—digestive system, metabolism, and enzymes—evolved from eating habits *over the course of millions of years*.

Even though we have gone through the most wondrous technical revolution the world has ever seen, we are still mammals. Nothing in our biology has changed in many, many millennia. We still give birth to

47

live offspring the same as all of our kind. We still have the same digestion. The mouth is still the place where the splitting of starches and sugars begins. And we're still governed by the laws of body chemistry.

Yet, we know more about refrigerators, televisions, and computers than about our closest companion: our body.

Well, you may say, our brain—a biochemical drug factory composed of the most flexible matter in our body—has developed and changed and adapted dramatically. This is true, but the brain didn't change dramatically within a couple of decades. It took thousands and thousands of years to evolve. Generally, it takes a millennium for our bodies to undergo really dramatic changes.

But, we asked our BioChemical Machine to change within several decades! Our body—which developed over the course of 200 million years—was supposed to adapt, within a relatively short space of time, to a radically changed world of supermarkets and fast food restaurants, where you just have to choose and your food is provided.

During the millions of years of mammalian development, there was no cooked meat or fish, no processed cheese, and no pasteurized and homogenized milk to bother anyone's body chemistry. There were only good proteins available, like those foods found in the "Neutral" column of the A&B Chart.

*At this point, I would like you to keep the BioChemical **A&B Chart** at hand. By glancing from time to time at this list, you will see that all food items are classified into three groups: "A", "B", or "Neutral" (that include good proteins).*

As you can see from the A&B Chart, "Neutrals" include not only salami, beef-salami, smoked and rolled ham, bacon, smoked sausages, beef jerky, smoked and marinated fish, beans, fava beans, lentils, all kinds of nuts, seeds, avocados, mushrooms, vegetables, salads, sprouts, olives, herbs, and blueberries—but also butter, oils, mayonnaise (no typo!), and a lot of dairy products, such as cream, heavy cream, sour cream, yogurt, whey, cottage cheese, mozzarella, Kefir, sheep's milk cheese (such as Roquefort), goat's milk cheese (such as feta), Camembert, cream Brie, cream Gouda, and other cheeses *above* 60% fat.

If eaten properly—which means according to the laws of your body chemistry—"Neutral" food items, even the often-vilified dairy products, butter, and oils, *do not* cause health and weight problems. The even bigger bonus: you can eat *anything and at any time* from the "Neutral" group; *24 hours a day, 7 days a week.*

Good Proteins Gone Bad

But first things first. Let's delve into the history of the problem— the birth of the bad proteins. We'll begin with the most common belief about our more recent ancestors, *Homo erectus*, and the excuse for making cooked meat a major part of our diet.

They were supposed to be wild killer apes that primarily ate meat and that's why we are, allegedly, still doing the same. But the truth is, at no time were we near being a meat-devouring ape, as falsely maintained by anthropologists for 27 years.[10]

Homo erectus was not primarily even a hunter. Both men and women hunted only from time to time. They were mostly simple and peaceful gatherers of vegetables, fruits, seeds, and nuts, who mainly cracked bones left behind by predatory animals in order to eat the marrow.[10] Marrow is not only a good protein, but it also contains the number one energy supplier: Fat.

For thousands of years, our ancestors ate foods like those found in the "A" and "Neutral" columns of the A&B Chart, which include good proteins such as smoked or rolled ham, legumes, cured and dried meat, salami, and smoked fish. There were no historically new, bad or extremely-bad proteins like those found in the "B" column of the A&B Chart such as low-fat or fat-free cheese, cooked meat, or cooked fish. Yet our ancestors' metabolism was satisfied. They got it all: carbohydrates, fats, and proteins. *Why?* Because most foods found in nature strike a consistent balance of carbohydrates, fats, and proteins.

So what makes a protein good or bad? When our ingenious ancestors invented the unique concept of cooking, it changed the nature of proteins. Every raw meat, fish, and milk and dairy product is "Neutral" by nature, creating no conflict within our body. The same is true for cured, dried, and smoked meat and fish.

It is the cooking process that changes (denatures) the chemistry of proteins, altering their sophisticated configuration/tertiary structure. Exposure to high temperatures changes the chemistry of good proteins and turns them into extremely-bad proteins that are so damaging to our health.

Our body chemistry, after only about a half century of eating this way, is still not adjusted to such hardship. Statistics like the 700% increase in U.S. diabetes cases over the last thirty years reflect this reality.[11]

Even our most recent ancestors, who domesticated animals and lived a very different life that included cooked meat—the extremely-bad proteins—didn't have the luxury of slaughtering one of their cows, goats, or sheep every day. Most people were poor and did not have several or even one animal. If they had livestock, it was reserved for festivals and special events. When an entire family or a village shared in the eating of one animal each person got only a very small piece.

If there was enough left over, they dried, smoked and cured the meat. For thousands of years our ancestors have eaten very little meat; most of it preserved. These preserved foods, however, are "Neutral" proteins the good proteins. This is why today's salami, rolled ham, pemmican (beef jerky), smoked bacon, and dried, smoked, or cured fish belong to the "Neutral" group. Rolled ham, for example, will be first cured and then stored in salt for three to four weeks. Afterwards, in order to ensure its durability, the ham will be dried and smoked, *but not cooked*. Other sausages, like salami, are made of uncooked muscle and fat but without adding water. They are preserved due to drying, smoking, or curing—NOT cooking. The same is valid for any smoked, dried, or cured food item.

At this point I would like to tell you about a real-life demonstration of the danger of extremely-bad protein consumption: In Tibet, it was once the custom not to immediately execute any person sentenced to death. The Tibetans wanted a true punishment for those who undermined their society. To that end, the incarcerated felon was fed *nothing but cooked meat.*

We don't eat a lot of extremely-bad protein because we have been sentenced to death; *we do it voluntarily.* We eat much more protein than is required for tissue

51

replacement. *Why?* During the 1950s and 1960s the rising meat industry hammered slogans like "Eat meat. It's good for your energy" into people's minds. Soon, nobody doubted that a big man needs a big steak if he wants to be strong. *But this is not the case.*

As paradoxical as it may sound, it is entirely possible to develop a protein deficiency while eating too much bad and extremely-bad proteins ("B" column on the A&B Charts). However, good proteins (middle column on the A&B Chart) are necessary for a healthy body, as well as fat, the #1 and carbohydrates, the #2 energy suppliers.

How can you learn the laws of your body chemistry if you hear, day in and day out, about all kinds of fairy tales about all kinds of foods by companies that have turned you into a money-making machine? Yet the real problem is not that companies want to make money; the real problem is that you are, unknowingly, poisoning yourself slowly but surely. Ironically, companies will *still* make sufficient money once people begin to eat according to the laws of body chemistry.

Our body chemistry cannot change overnight. We need to find a solution to deal with the current reality; one that adjusts our modern eating habits to our old-fashioned digestive chemistry. And that's what the A&B Method is all about.

Let's take human milk as an example of how Mother Nature meant us to eat. Human breast milk is approximately 85% water. The remainder is 6.9% carbohydrates, 3.7% fat, and 1.2% protein. We all know that there is no better food in this world than mother's milk for the first year of life.

This ratio is indeed interesting, because human milk is made up of the best energy suppliers: carbohydrates and fats. Only a small percentage of the milk is protein. In the final analysis, this ratio is exactly Mother Nature's concept for our eating habits.

What did the majority of our ancestors really do with their cows, goats, or sheep over the last 10,000 years? They drank the milk and produced (but did not pasteurize and homogenize) healthy dairy products like butter, cream, sour cream, buttermilk, all kind of curds (like the curdled cheese that we call today cottage cheese), and goat's or sheep's milk cheese (like feta)—that are all good protein sources.

Cow's milk would be "Neutral" in its original state. That's why our ancestors ate compatibly by eating bread and drinking milk and milk products—thus "A" and "Neutral". The pasteurizing and homogenizing process changes the chemistry of milk, so today it falls into the "B" column on the A&B Chart. But despite pasteurizing and homogenizing, (which means eating denatured protein), milk is still a moderate base-builder; a healthy, acid-nullifying food *if* ingested with compatible foods from the "B" column; especially apples and other "B" fruits, and, of course, with "Neutrals".

However, some dairy products are unhealthy acid-builders. Cheeses, which are below 50% fat like those found in the "B" column are recent inventions, thus *new history*. Our factories and methods of processing the new history foods became more sophisticated—and so did our cheese. It became a bad protein.

53

> **BioChemical Machine Fact:** *Modern food processing has had the same effects on carbohydrates like refined flour products and white-polished rice, as well as fats like hardened margarine. I want to emphasize that although new history foods are unhealthy acid-builders; their impact on health is not nearly as damaging as the extremely-bad proteins.*

As you will read throughout the book, the bad and extremely-bad proteins are emergency suppliers to our metabolism. By relying on *either* protein you will be satiated for the moment, especially at the beginning of dieting, but will soon be very hungry as it is a very poor fuel on which to support activity—expensive in every sense of the word. Yet it is no secret that almost every fad diet is based on too much of these bad and extremely-bad proteins. That's why fad diets leave you hungry.

You are not hungry because you decided to lose weight or because you are too weak to control your cravings (which leads to feelings of guilt). You are hungry because you and your metabolism *are,* in fact, starving. Hunger is a signal, a chemical reaction that your body isn't getting what your metabolism needs to do its job: minerals, amino acids, fatty acids, enzymes, fats, carbohydrates, and a small amount of good proteins from the "Neutral" group on the A&B Chart.

Yet, there are sufficient sources which will provide you with healthy protein, such as wheat bread, rye bread, brown rice, and, of course, base-builders such as fruits, vegetables, and salads. Ironically, the best and most high-grade protein is nowhere else but in the potato!

> **BioChemical Machine Fact:** *The idea of "calories" stems from the time when the steam engine was born: put in coal and out comes energy. Unfortunately, today, diet gurus would have us believe that it must be the same with food. One calorie is the unit of heat that is required to warm 1 gram of water from 14.5 to 15.5 degrees Celsius. That's all. It's just a measurement of heat.* **We are not steamboats;** *we are a more complicated BioChemical Machine, which adheres to the laws of our body's own chemistry.* **With the BioChemical A&B Method, you do NOT need to count calories**.

And here we are. We arc at the beginning of the journey that could change your life forever. The BioChemical A&B Method will realign your body chemistry to the modern world. It is the perfect match of food chemistry and body chemistry. By following the principles of the BioChemical A&B Method, you will make a dramatic, fast, and long-term difference in your overall well-being. You will feel the difference within the first two weeks—its impact is that powerful. Your vitality will begin to return and heartburn, which is the direct result of excessive stomach acid in the lower esophagus, will start to disappear.

This immediate success is not as much astonishing as it is logical. As your unbalanced body chemistry begins to regulate itself, step-by-step your body will be able to get rid of the poisons you have accumulated and stored up; probably over the course of many years.

The next chapter will give you a clearer picture why the perfect match of body chemistry and food chemistry—and the knowledge that two different types of digestion exist for protein is of such great significance, and how this match will ensure you never poison yourself again. With the BioChemical A&B Method, your body will never return to a hyper-acidic state, but will instead maintain the vital *alkaline reserve.*

Therefore, let us discuss the cause of Self-Poisoning: The Alkaline Deficit and its impact on our health, energy, and body weight...because *It's Not About Food—It's About Your Cells.*

Throughout the book you will read about good protein turned bad, i.e., that cooked, fried or grilled meat is bad protein. This does NOT mean that you may no longer eat meat in the frame of the BioChemical A&B Method (unless you are ill and will do LEVEL TWO—eating meat moderately—see Chapter 19 and 20). On the contrary, you can eat meat, chicken and steak— but you will learn to eat it the BioChemical A&B way so that it will NOT harm your BioChemical Machine. Chicken, steak or any other "B" meat can be eaten with anything from "B" and "Neutral" groups (which includes the good proteins). Just for example: chicken with oranges (tastes delicious!), and/or with vegetables, and/or salads, and/or sour cream sauce and so many other things...

Also, throughout The BioChemical Machine, *you will read the term "uncooked meat." Do not interpret this as a recommendation to eat raw meat. It simply refers to any method of cooking meats that does not employ the protein damaging temperatures associated with traditional ovens and stovetop cooking. There are numerous other methods for healthful meat preparation, such as curing, drying, and smoking.*

Chapter 2

IT'S NOT ABOUT FOOD—IT'S ABOUT YOUR CELLS:
A Road to Self-Poisoning

I am always astonished to hear people talking about guilt in connection with dieting and its relapse. *How can anyone feel guilty about the desire to eat?* Eating is one of the five basic human needs, along with drinking, breathing, sleeping, and sex. How can anyone feel guilty about something that is stronger than our will? We are born with the desire to eat in order to live. No basic human need would ever create any problem for us as long as it didn't interfere with Mother Nature. But this is what we have done, and not only when it comes to food.

If anyone is "guilty," then it's our industrial revolution and prosperity itself. Do you want to blame yourself for the rise of the food industry and its seductive products? New food products require a new approach to matching food chemistry and body chemistry.

This new approach is crucial in dealing with all those alluring products found in supermarkets and restaurants. *We cannot turn back the clock. The food industry is part of our world—and we can learn to live in it in a way that leaves us healthy and energetic.*

The Cell—Understanding the Problem

Our very existence is based on the cell.* If our cells are not healthy; we are not healthy. Our organs require healthy cells to function perfectly. The food we eat is responsible for the nourishment of our cells. Thus, we can decide the health of our cells and ourselves by eating according to the laws of our body chemistry.

But here's the catch: most people don't know about the perfect match of food and body chemistry and the fact that there are two different types of digestion that exist for proteins—one for the good proteins (pure/high grade protein), another for bad proteins (abnormal proteins). Therefore, people unknowingly disregard the laws of chemistry, build up acid after acid, and poison themselves. If you poison your body over many years by not eating correctly, you can almost be sure that you will develop serious illnesses later in life.

Fatigue is often the *first indication* that something is wrong with our cells and thus, our body chemistry. One-third of the U.S. population has difficulty staying awake after eating.[12] Often, the causes of fatigue are also harbingers of more serious problems. What's more, pathological fatigue is only *one result* of unknowingly poisoning yourself. Step by step, additional physical symptoms will arise; coughing, headaches, swollen eyelids, dizziness, bloodshot eyes, and cloudy vision.

---

*The cell, in biology, is a discrete, membrane-bound portion of living matter. It is the smallest unit capable of an independent existence. All living organisms consist of one or more cells, with the exception of viruses.

But this is *just the beginning*. Starting around age thirty, human cell activity begins to slow and the regeneration process declines decade by decade. The immune system reduces its production of antibodies, leaving us more susceptible to sickness. Muscle mass is replaced by fat unless we do something about it.

One day you will come to the point that it feels as if your body is falling apart. Probably you will pacify yourself with the common belief that pain after fifty is the fate of every human being on earth. But this is just not true. Once you know how to match food and body chemistry, you will have control over your health and energy and slow down the aging process. You will not only have more fun during your early and middle years, but also really look forward to your "golden" years. As Dr. Hay says, "it is more a question of understanding foods and…at the same time respecting the laws of chemistry."[14]

Remember! If your cells are healthy, *you are healthy*. The food we eat and how we eat it makes all the difference. You will maximize the efficiency of your digestive system, which in turn will help maintain properly functioning metabolism. A strong metabolism will ensure that you will not be storing poisonous cells with acidic end products. A healthy metabolism is also vital for your immune system; the decline of the metabolism creates a higher risk for infection and, ultimately, chronic diseases. "Disease never attacks healthy tissue; for the resistant body will not harbor infection, as it will not degenerate in structure and function," Dr. Quazi Al Tariq says.

A very, very sad statistic reflects this fact: "100,000 Americans will die [each year] because of wrong dieting."[3]

I began pondering the image of food. Food: what an ordinary thing. Even haute cuisine doesn't have the glamour of Cartier, Gucci, or Chanel. But without it you couldn't even think of Cartier, Gucci, and Chanel. *Think about it.* If we are arrogant in regard to our basic nature, we are poisoning ourselves. Did I say arrogant? Perhaps I should say ignorant, because we *would* respect our basic nature if we understood it. No one would voluntarily poison him or herself, creating a never-ending struggle with weight problems, chronic disease, pain, and even an early death.

This book is the instruction manual for the way your body—your BioChemical Machine—interacts with food. It's *complicated* if you don't know the laws of your body's chemistry; *simple* once you do.

Therefore, let's talk about the underlying cause of so many problems relating to our health.

What Causes Self-Poisoning?

"Self-poisoning" goes by many names: over-acidification, toxification, toxemia, self-toxification, or intoxification. But all refer to the acidic end products of digestion and metabolism; your body's toxic waste.

There are TWO different ways your body creates this toxic waste: One that we *cannot* control and *one* that we can:

1. THE NORMAL PROCESS OF METABOLISM:
    Many of the billions of cells that make up our
    bodies die every day. They are constantly being
    replaced by new cells. The dead cells must be
    removed by one of our excretory organs: lungs,
    bowels, skin, liver, or kidneys as quickly as
    possible. A certain amount of these acidic end
    products are the result of the body's own
    decomposition and death. It is during this
    replacement process that the *acidic debris* of
    dying cells accumulates in the body.

2. DISREGARDING BODY CHEMISTRY: If you
    burden your metabolism by eating *incompatible*
    foods that disregard the laws of your body
    chemistry, you are producing a surplus of
    poisonous cells that can't be excreted fast enough
    or incorporated into cell structures. This creates
    an accumulation of debilitating poisons in your
    system.

Many, if not most illnesses, are related to the surplus
of these metabolic-related toxic wastes that remain
somewhere in your body instead of being eliminated
through the skin, colon, liver, and kidneys. The tissue
residues determine illness or health. Disease rarely
develops in normal tissues; those nourished with a
proper blood supply and, thus, a higher degree of
alkalinity.

The blood works according to very narrow parameters and sickness can quickly result if these parameters are not respected. "The blood, if not toxin-free, puts a tremendous strain upon the heart," says Dr. Al Tariq.[15] The same happens to be the case with the liver, lungs, pancreas, kidneys, thyroid gland, adrenal glands, and lymphatic system. Acid waste almost always reaches the tissues through blood and lymph toxicity.

> *BioChemical Machine Fact:* *Body chemistry is not negotiable. It must be respected in order to remain healthy, energetic, and free of pain. Your alkaline reserve makes the difference.*

The Alkaline Reserve

I'm sure that many of you will ask the question "Why don't we immediately die from self-poisoning?" The answer is simple. We are a vigorous species meant to survive. We are a biological masterpiece. Mother Nature allowed us to evolve from one single cell into hundreds of billions of cells. We limit ourselves by interfering with Mother Nature and her concept of our body chemistry.

In reality, it is a miracle that we are able to survive our modern eating habits while almost completely disregarding the laws of body chemistry. To make this miracle happen, Mother Nature equipped us with a safety net; a buffer system that makes the necessary adjustments.

"The alkaline* reserve acts as a buffer to maintain proper balance in the blood," explains Dr. Al Tariq.[16] This buffer is a mixture of chemical compounds chosen to maintain a steady pH** (the scale for measuring acidity or alkalinity).

There are several different buffer systems in our body and several organs have the capacity to provide them. The most common buffers consist of a weak organic acid and a mixture of salts of phosphoric acids. The addition of either an acid or a base causes a shift in the chemical equilibrium, thus keeping the pH constant.

Scientists began studying and quantifying the importance of the alkaline reserve in the laboratory to more fully understand the fluctuations of the content of CO_2 and HCO_3 in the blood. They documented the importance of this bicarbonate system. Further buffer systems in the blood are proteins and inorganic phosphates. Lungs and kidneys also provide buffer capacity. Blood, lungs, and kidneys compensate for disturbances in the acid-alkaline balance of a healthy person. This is the way we are able to adapt to extreme situations, which we all do; day in and day out.

---

*ALKALINE: in our context, a substance having a pH above that of neutral water (7.0) when in solution. Signified as pH (potential of hydrogen), alkaline fluids, such as the blood (pH about 7.4), have the ability to neutralize acids (solutions below pH 7.0). Metabolic wastes are acids, and the alkaline reserve of the blood neutralizes them until they are excreted (Medical Dictionary).

**pH is the scale for measuring acidity or alkalinity. "From the standpoint of pure energy, pH is the measurement of electrical resistance between negative and positive ions in the body. The pH level is a measurement of the number of hydroxyl (OH-) ions which are negative and alkaline-forming, as opposed to the amount of hydrogen (H+) ions that are positive and acid-forming. Alkaline and acid-forming reactions are purely electro-chemical—i.e., pH measures how much the negative (alkaline-forming) ions and positive (acid-forming) ions push against one another," explains Dr. Al Tariq.[20]

But even buffer systems have their limit if we overburden our metabolism by disregarding the laws of our body's chemistry. The alkaline reserve is only a back-up system with limited capacity to keep you from constantly poisoning yourself. *

BioChemical Machine Fact: *Chronic alkaline deficit is a major reason for getting sick. Fatigue is the first sign that something is wrong with our body chemistry. But it also applies the other way around—when self-poisoning is gone then fatigue is gone.*

"The function of every organ and tissue depends on the height, breadth, and depth of the alkaline reserve," explains Dr. Al Tariq.[17] "The lower the alkaline level, the lower the function. Conversely, the higher the alkaline reserve, the higher the level of activity our bodies can perform. The alkaline reserve is the body's bank account."[18]

I would add that it's more than a bank account; maybe better described as a savings account that the body can call upon anytime to release alkaline elements to neutralize harmful acids; but there's a limit to how much can be saved. Since most people don't know this fact, they attempt to function with deficient alkaline reserves.

---

*Once, the scientific community believed that the body maintains its acid-alkaline balance through the buffer systems. It was believed that excessive carbonic acid would be exhaled through the lungs and the kidneys would release the remaining acids directly; or in the form of easily soluble salts. Contemporary scientists proved the existence of the phenomenon—which is self-poisoning.

The Alkaline Deficit

Therefore, let's talk about the *corpus delicti*...the cause for most of our problems: "The Alkaline Deficit", which was the result of Dr. Hay's revolutionary research about the acid-alkaline balance and alkaline reserve. Acid and alkaline are opposites that should be balanced. You should have neither too much alkaline in your blood nor too much acid. The alkaline reserve ensures that your body will be able to maintain this balance. It is responsible for binding these acids as they form and will decide how we live; even whether we live at all.

But what are acids? Are acids really as bad as described throughout this chapter? If we're talking about unhealthy acids...then the answer is yes. But we need to distinguish between healthy and unhealthy acids because, indeed there are acids your body needs; acids that are vital to good health:

STOMACH ACIDITY
Hydrochloric acid (HCl) is produced by the stomach to digest foods. It is an essential acid that is produced by our body as a natural process. Digestion produces stomach acids. All other acids are products of metabolism.

THE HEALTHY METABOLIC ACIDS
By nature, our body needs small portions of acid-building foods in order to fulfill certain tasks. For example: acid causes pain on the free nerve endings as an important warning signal. Pain indicates that something is wrong with our body. Lactic acid and carbon dioxide originate in hardworking muscles and

create the fatigue that warns us about excessive physical activity. The increase of carbon dioxide levels in the blood affects the way we breathe so that more carbon dioxide will be exhaled through deeper breathing to restore the acid-alkaline balance.

THE UNHEALTHY METABOLIC ACIDS
The unhealthy acids, the cause of the alkaline deficit, are created by disregarding the A&B principles and eating too much of the bad and extremely-bad proteins. The right consumption amount is different for everyone. Healthy, active individuals should have no difficulties properly metabolizing these proteins. However, individuals suffering from serious health ailments must limit consumption of bad and extremely-bad proteins— shaded gray and red on the A&B Chart LEVEL TWO— and denatured carbohydrates group III—shaded gray on the A&B Chart LEVEL TWO—to once a month and then only along with raw, fresh base-builders. You will read much more about this in subsequent chapters.

The Solution

But what is the solution to restoring your body's alkaline savings account? It's simple: smart dietary habits that build up and sustain an alkaline reserve. The only way alkaline and acid enter your body is by eating. Some foods will be metabolized into alkaline and others into acid. If you don't eat according to the laws of your body chemistry, your BioChemical Machine will undergo undue hardship and eventually be "out of order." In other words: fatigued; in pain; or ill.

I'm sure you will say, "You make it sound so easy, but seductive foods in every supermarket, deli, and fast food restaurant are just lurking around every corner inviting me to eat and eat and eat. Who in the world can think of acid or alkaline when their mouth is watering?" You are right. This is the dilemma of our modern world. But if you take a close look at the A&B Chart (LEVEL ONE for healthy people and LEVEL TWO for ill people) you'll see that you can eat *almost anything* you want—PROVIDED you match foods according to their chemical compatibility with your body.*

LEVEL ONE
The first important step is to eat according to the BioChemical A&B Method—the perfect match of food chemistry and body chemistry. Following these principles will make the quickest and largest difference.

LEVEL TWO
People with health problems need to, not only eat according to the BioChemical A&B Method (LEVEL ONE), but also follow the 80% base-builders/20% healthy acid-builders ratio (LEVEL TWO)—avoiding, if not eliminating, the bad and extremely-bad proteins from their diet.

---

*Although the difference between acidosis and alkalosis seems to be very slight (as measured in terms of pH), this difference is vital to good health, energy, and weight control. Even a latent over-acidification of tissues with still normal alkaline reserve and normal acid-alkaline balance can pave the way for many illnesses.[19]

By following the BioChemical A&B Method, you'll bring your weight under control, curtailing the effects of obesity, which brings with it a host of health nightmares. Obesity is linked to numerous disturbances of the metabolism, such as increased fat levels in the blood, kidney stones, diabetes, varicose veins, disturbances of the blood circulation, and the risk of developing thrombosis and embolism. Excessive weight also burdens the spinal column and the hip and knee joints. It is well known that obesity is a risk factor for heart and circulatory diseases and for breast and colon cancer. Eventually, it leads to a more frequent appearance of various forms of cancer.*

Knowledge is power. And knowledge of yourself means that you will have control over your health, weight, energy, and even over the speed of your aging process. Armed with the knowledge about the perfect match of food chemistry and body chemistry and its creation of the vital acid-alkaline balance, you will know what is right and what is wrong for your body. You don't need to study medicine or biochemistry in order to understand how your body works. The A&B Chart makes it easy to follow the principles of your body chemistry and to turn knowledge into practice. It's just a question of becoming conscious that we are a BioChemical Machine that needs to be carefully treated.

---

*In December 1998 the NBC show interviewed John J. Lynch of the American Cancer Society, who stated that "wrong diet was responsible for 40% of the cancer cases."[21] The American Cancer Society published in "Cancer Prevention & Early Detection," © 2000: "According to scientific research done over the past two decades, about one-third of all US cancer deaths can be attributed to the adult diet, including its effect on obesity."

As a side effect, many health and weight problems will simply disappear.

What did Dr. Hay say a hundred years ago? "When intoxification is gone then fatigue is gone...." When fatigue is gone; energy is back. And when energy is back; health is back. Nothing has changed since Dr. Hay's revolutionary discovery. This was the reality 200 million years ago, a hundred years ago, and it is valid for the six billion people who live today on this wonderful planet. It will be the reality as long as humans exist. No diet drink, no low-carb or high-protein diet, no glycemic index, no diet bar, no caloric counting, and no "abracadabra" promises can satisfy your metabolism. Why? Because our organs and glands function properly in exact proportion to the amount of alkaline and acid levels in the system. Yet we are still running after the mirage that any fad diet or miracle pill could satisfy such a sophisticated machine like ours.

In Chapter 3, you'll learn more about how your sophisticated BioChemical Machine operates.

PART II

THE BIOCHEMICAL A&B METHOD PRINCIPLES

Balancing The BioChemical Machine

Chapter 3

THE BIOCHEMICAL MACHINE
The Key Factor to Eliminate Weight and Health Problems: Understanding the two different types of protein digestion

Self-poisoning does not occur overnight. It takes years, if not decades of making bad choices to build up poison in our BioChemical Machine. Unfortunately, we don't immediately feel the extent of the damage because our species is equipped to survive. On the one hand this is fortunate; on the other, that's exactly where the danger lies. If we immediately became ill when we ate incorrectly, we would quickly learn to always eat right.

Our body has a tremendous power to correct itself. This correction begins with the food we eat. At the heart of your body's delicate biochemical balance is food and the way it is digested. As the distribution center of your well-being, digestion nourishes cells and therefore tissues, the lymphatic system, and all organs. The cells and liver produce enzymes and supply blood with all needed substances.

Without digestion there is no energy. And without energy there is no life. In short, digestion is the center of your very existence.

Gaining control over your digestion can change your life forever. It empowers your metabolism to do a proper and efficient job enabling it to cleanse your body of poisoned cells and acidic end products. So understanding the digestive process is an important starting point.

Let's begin by examining the different ways your body digests different foods—and why foods are categorized the way they are on the A&B Chart.

1. GOOD PROTEIN DIGESTION
"Neutral" Column

"Neutral" proteins—the foods found in the middle column of the BioChemical A&B Chart such as uncooked meats, fish (smoked, cured, etc.), and dairy products that have not been homogenized or pasteurized, as well as uncooked or cooked egg yolks— are "old history"; so much a part of our biological nature through the millennia that your body has *no trouble* digesting them. They can be eaten at any time with foods from the "A" *or* "B" column or any other item in the "Neutral" group on the A&B Chart.

2. BAD PROTEIN DIGESTION
"B" Column

Extremely-bad and bad proteins like those found in the "B" column of the BioChemical A&B Chart are easy to digest PROVIDED you don't ask your body to do so with other foods from the "A" column at the same time.

Digestion of the "new history" foods; "B" proteins like cooked meats, eggs, cheeses below 50% fat, and pasteurized and homogenized milk causes acid to build up in your body—that you now know, deduct from the important alkaline reserve. But as long as you don't eat incompatible foods, as defined by the A&B Chart, your body can cope.

To make the digestion of "B" proteins (the historically new, bad and extremely-bad proteins) possible, the stomach's gastric juices need to be very acidic. "B" protein digestion begins in the stomach with an enzyme, called pepsin, in the presence of hydrochloric acid. Without the action of pepsin, those acid-building "B" proteins couldn't go through the first step of digestion.

BioChemical Machine Fact: *The enzyme pepsin will act only in an acidic environment.*

It's during this first step that "B" proteins are reduced to amino acids and peptides. However, starches (complex carbohydrates), sugars, and fats are not digested by these gastric juices. The second step in this digestion process takes place in the small intestine. It's there that the "B" protein digestive process is completed by pancreatic juice, intestinal juice, and bile. The pancreatic juice contains the enzymes trypsin, amylase, and lipase that are vital to completing this process.

2. CARBOHYDRATE DIGESTION
"A" Column

Unlike the acid-building "B" proteins, carbohydrates must have alkaline conditions to be digested.

Chewing is the first and foremost, underrated step in digesting carbohydrates. In addition to the fact that digestive juices can react more easily to finer particles of food, saliva is essential to breaking down carbohydrates. *Why?* Saliva contains an enzyme called amylase; its role is to split the complex carbohydrate and sugars into smaller units or simple sugars.

BioChemical Machine Fact: The enzyme amylase will act only in a positive alkaline environment.

After the food is swallowed it passes through the esophagus into the stomach where it mixes with abdominal amylase and is reduced into simple sugars; ready for intestinal digestion. If the environment isn't at least slightly alkaline—digestion will be hindered and starches will reach the small intestine almost undigested.

Digestion continues in the small intestine where additional amylase, generated from the pancreas and secreted from the walls of the small intestine, decompose the remaining starches into simple sugars.

Again, if the environment of the small intestine isn't slightly alkaline allowing the amylase to do its work; digestion will be hindered. One consequence is a buildup of gases, which causes the infamous feeling of fullness, fatigue, and pain.

BioChemical Machine Fact: The enzymes pepsin (required for bad and extremely-bad protein digestion) and amylase (required for carbohydrate digestion) inhibit each other's action when put together.

By eating different types of foods that require two different types of digestion ("A" and "B" columns at the same time), we make it difficult for our bodies to efficiently digest food. We are also creating a chaotic situation for the mixing chamber—the stomach. The stomach cannot be both acidic and alkaline at the same time. As stated before, the enzyme amylase can function only if sufficient alkaline is available. Without the stimulation of this alkaline medium there is no action of the enzyme amylase on carbohydrates. Even the slightest acid reaction can slow down the splitting process of carbohydrates and can go so far as to *arrest* the process of starch breakdown.

When we eat chemically incompatible foods together, digestion is not only made more difficult but is considerably delayed. We may even make it impossible to digest the foods completely. As stated before, when we put conflicting enzymes together during the digestive process they are unable to function properly.

3. FAT DIGESTION
"Neutral" Column

Advertisers have invested huge sums of money and time into making you believe the slogan "fat makes fat." This fallacy has become big business in regard to your health. The truth is, because of their chemical makeup, all fats and oils fall under the "Neutral" category on the BioChemical A&B Chart.

Unlike "B" proteins and carbohydrates, fats and oils don't require special treatment to prepare them for digestion in the small intestine.

Although the stomach and small intestine secrete fat-decomposing enzymes—their significance is small.

The pancreas does most of the work by secreting the enzyme pancreas-lipase into the duodenum, where, with the help of liver-produced bile, the fats are broken down and emulsified into a soapy form and easily absorbed into the bloodstream. To further support the metabolic breakdown of fats always eat foods that contain healthy supplies of pantothenic acid. Pantothenic acid is a vitamin that plays a central role in fat breakdown. Pantothenic acid is available in vegetables, especially cauliflower (which detoxifies cells and creates new skin) and mushrooms, but it is also found in whole wheat bread, nuts, and yeast.

Now that you have a better understanding of how certain foods are digested differently, let's examine how we can utilize this knowledge to properly balance your BioChemical Machine.

Chapter 4

THE BIOCHEMICAL
A&B CHARTS:
LEVEL ONE & LEVEL TWO
Healthy Living Without Diets

Dispense with the magic pills promising a quick fix, the fad diets that don't work, and the deprivation that leaves you hungry and unhappy. The BioChemical A&B Method is about what you should eat based on your body chemistry.

The A&B Method is all about learning how to contend with, and even reverse, the health-damaging effects caused by the "new history" food items: bad and extremely-bad proteins. As discussed earlier, this group of proteins is responsible for most—if not all—health and weight problems because they create excessive acidity, thereby reducing the effectiveness of digestive enzymes and ultimately undermining your alkaline reserve. If you choose foods based on their compatibility, then your BioChemical Machine will be kept in perfect balance and you will enjoy all the benefits of good health.

The BioChemical A&B Chart was developed to give you all the information you need to make the right choices based on your physical condition. Everyone is different. That's why I created two A&B Charts: LEVEL ONE for healthy people. LEVEL TWO for people with health problems, obesity, and those who care for prevention. How you use the A&B Chart will depend on different factors: age, weight, and current health. If you are at your ideal weight and in good health, you can eat virtually anything you want, PROVIDED you match foods according to their chemical compatibility: 24/7 "Neutrals" (that includes the good proteins), "A" column with "Neutral"; "B" column with "Neutral", *but never foods from the "A" and "B" column together at the same meal.*

Base-Builder or Acid-Builder?
It's as Easy as Yellow, White, Gray, and Red

In LEVEL TWO of the BioChemical A&B Method, the foods under each column on the A&B Chart are shaded yellow, white, gray, or red. This was done to help you distinguish between foods that are base-builders and those that are acid-builders. If you have health problems, then you need to pay special attention to the color coordination on the LEVEL TWO A&B Chart. In addition to following the principles behind the "A", "B", and "Neutral" columns, you will also want to choose foods that create a diet balanced of 80% base-builders to 20% **healthy** acid-builders.

A good rule of thumb to remember is:
Eat plenty from the YELLOW.
Eat moderately from the WHITE.
Avoid the GRAY and RED as much as possible.

YELLOW: Very Healthy Base-Builders

The foods you find shaded yellow on the BioChemical A&B Chart are the strong and moderate base-builders that should make up the backbone of your diet. The strong base-builders are vital for your alkaline reserves and should be the major component of each day's menu, although moderate base-builders are still strong enough to increase alkalinity. Like strong base-builders, the moderates may be part of each day's base-building foods.

WHITE: Healthy Acid-Builders

Moderate acid-builders are the acid-builders that your body needs; ideally eaten *together* with base-builders. Remember...not *all* acids are bad. Your body needs small portions of certain acid-building foods in order to fulfill important tasks.

GRAY & RED: Unhealthy Acid-Builders

The "new history" foods are the **unhealthy** acid-builders. The way in which they are processed and prepared have made them bad, bad, bad and we *could* live without them—if they didn't taste so good! Some of these acid-builders are more damaging than others. They are the cooked meats shaded red under the "B" column. If you are in good health your body can absorb the costs of eating the occasional hamburger but, if you are suffering from any illness, the cost to your body chemistry really isn't worth it. So try not to eat too much of these **unhealthy** acid-builders especially the extremely-bad proteins from the "B" column which are the *worst* of the worst. If you *do* choose to eat from the gray or red group—religiously follow the A&B principles and eat them with strong base-builders such as fruits, vegetables, and salads.

Learning to Live With ALL Foods

As you can see, carbohydrates, proteins, and fats are found in all columns of both the LEVEL ONE and LEVEL TWO programs, as well as in each of the yellow, white, gray, and red color schemes. Gurus that demand you eliminate fat or carbohydrates from your diet to lose weight are simply wrong! All the food groups—carbohydrates, fats, and proteins—are valuable parts of a balanced diet, provided you abide by the A&B principles, that distinguish between the good and the bad in each.

For example: carbohydrates shaded yellow on the A&B Chart, such as potatoes, kale, millet, honey, sprouted grains, bananas, grapes, fresh figs, fresh dates, dried apples, dried plums, dried figs, dried dates, and raisins are excellent base-builders. They are very healthy and may be eaten *without limit*.

BioChemical Machine Fact: Conventional wisdom has maintained that eating potatoes is a bad idea if you're trying to lose weight. **Not so!** *Rich in vitamin and mineral content and packed with high-grade protein that provides essential amino acids, the potato is a strong base-builder and may be—even* **should be**—*eaten as often as possible. As long as you abide by the BioChemical A&B principles you may eat potatoes to your heart's content.*

However, not all carbohydrates are base-builders. Take for example natural, but *processed* carbohydrates like whole wheat bread. Our bread is refined and cooked or heated at temperatures above 300 degrees Fahrenheit changing it from a strong base-builder into a moderate acid-builder (at the boundary of being a moderate base-builder).[22] However, meat cooked at this temperature would turn it into an extremely-bad protein. These modern preparations cause the oxidation of wheat bread, which is why it releases carbonic acid into your system. Although it is relatively little acid in comparison to the following group, it should be eaten in the right proportion *with fresh base-builders.*

The same oxidation is true for grains such as natural rice, rye, oats, and corn, all of which are rich in vitamins and minerals. If compatibly eaten, they are also definitely a most healthy choice. As such, you'll find them— along with whole wheat bread—included in the white group on the LEVEL TWO A&B Chart.

Not All Carbohydrates are Created Equal

But not all carbohydrates are good for you. Unnatural or denatured carbohydrates and radically altered grains, like refined white flour and processed sugar, are strong acid-builders. When these concentrated carbohydrates are metabolized, large amounts of carbonic acid are released into the body (although their debris is not as toxic as the bad and extremely-bad proteins).

They, of course, are the carbohydrates shaded gray on the LEVEL TWO A&B Chart.

Healthy people may eat moderately from this group as long as they follow the principles behind the "A", "B", and "Neutral" columns. However, if you are struggling with health problems, eating foods from the gray group should be a rare occurrence.

BioChemical Machine Fact: You need five to ten times the quantity of white bread (as compared with whole wheat bread) just to feel satiated. White bread has no substantial food value. In the final analysis, it is more expensive than whole wheat bread.

As we explore throughout the book it becomes more obvious that when we eat natural foods in their natural forms we are not troubled with acid formation. Nature balances these foods very nicely for our digestive abilities and keeps our body chemistry in harmony.

It is when we diverge from what nature intended that we upset the balance of our BioChemical Machine and poison ourselves; gradually and unintentionally.

We don't need to starve our body of the right foods, causing health and weight problems, because we have the power to choose correctly. By following the BioChemical A&B Method, guided by LEVEL ONE or LEVEL TWO of the BioChemical A&B Chart you're on your way to perfect body chemistry and good health.

Chapter 5

THE BIG SEVEN ESSENTIALS
*Balancing Body Chemistry
for Health and Perfect Weight*

Now that you have an understanding of how your body chemistry reacts to different foods, let's get down to ways you can beneficially use this information. In this chapter, I've distilled the essence of the BioChemical A&B Method into seven essential steps. By incorporating these seven essentials into your day-to-day life, you'll *immediately* feel better and have more energy. You'll gain control of your appetite. Heartburn will disappear. In the long term, serious health and weight problems will improve and you'll even slow the aging process.

Is it really this simple? It *can* be, because your body chemistry is comprehensible, but not negotiable.

Essential #1
Learn How to Cope with the Bad
and Extremely-bad Proteins

"Neutrals" can be eaten at any time, *24 hours a day, 7 days a week*. But don't eat foods from the "B" group with foods from the "A" group because your BioChemical machinery is just not made for it! This is the fundamental principle of the BioChemical A&B Method and the key to a healthy and energetic life.

Eliminating the practice of eating foods from both the "A" column and "B" column during the same meals will result in an immediate boost to your alkaline reserve. In many cases, people have experienced the benefits within the first two weeks! This simple adjustment of your eating habits increases the effectiveness of your metabolism and jump-starts the process of cleansing your body of poisonous dead cells.

Essential #2
Replace Bad Proteins
with Healthy Good Proteins

All proteins are not created equal. As discussed, consuming excess amounts of the acid-building bad and extremely-bad "B" proteins is the likely cause of many of today's health problems. When cooked, foods from the "B" column leave behind *the greatest amount* of the most irritating debris in your body; a wide array of very acidic and very irritating salts; predominantly uric acid. Urea and uric acid remain in the body up to the time of excretion through the kidneys.

These two acids shift the acid-base balance toward an acidic (poisonous). At this stage, your body simply requires time to excrete the acid surplus.

However, as you know from Chapter 3, if your body is contending with digesting foods from both the "A" and "B" columns at the same time, you are putting an unnecessary burden on the buffer system—your alkaline reserve. As such, the body cannot excrete the acid surplus because the blood is unable to buffer the masses of accrued acids coming in waves. This build-up of acids causes self-poisoning and leads to the host of health problems I've discussed.

The BioChemical A&B Chart will help you distinguish between good and bad and extremely-bad proteins:

> **GOOD PROTEINS:** The healthy proteins—found in the "Neutral" middle column of the BioChemical A&B Chart and highlighted in white and yellow.

> **BAD & EXTREMELY-BAD PROTEINS:** The unhealthy proteins—found in the "B" column of the BioChemical A&B Chart and highlighted in gray and red.

Don't be confused that whole milk is included in the "B" column. Despite the fact that milk is a moderate base-builder (boosting the alkaline reserve) it is still healthy. Originally, whole milk was a very strong base-builder and belonged to the "Neutrals", but modern pasteurizing and homogenizing changed the chemistry of milk. So, we should no longer drink milk along with foods from the "A" column of the BioChemical A&B Chart, such as bread or potatoes. However, whole milk is still one of the best foods to detoxify the body in the morning.

And, despite pasteurizing, milk remains a moderate base-builder and a good source of protein. What's more, increasing numbers of supermarkets are selling whole milk that is free of hormones and unnecessary chemicals.

What are the results of eating bad and extremely-bad proteins? As an example, let's take the diseases osteoporosis and arthritis. Remember that strong acid-building food, like cooked meat, shifts the pH balance in the body towards an acidic balance. If the body cannot buffer the acid in its blood, it will take vital minerals from the bones. The body is forced to mobilize calcium, magnesium, and potassium from its reserves to balance the bases and acids in the blood and cells. Over time, over-acidification of the blood can lead to the degeneration of the bones.

Even though the body has vital alkaline reserves that neutralize acids, the fewer acids we create, the fewer bases we withdraw from our body's alkaline reserves. Eating too many bad and extremely-bad proteins drains our alkaline reserves.

Essential #3
Eat More of the Right Food:
Base-Builders and Healthy Carbohydrates

Your food choices should be rich with the right kinds of food that you'll find highlighted in white and yellow on all three columns of the BioChemical A&B Chart. Good proteins can be eaten 24/7. The only exception to this would be for those following LEVEL TWO where 80% of the food must be **FRESH** base-builders. Healthy, good proteins are highlighted in white and yellow on the "Neutral" column of the BioChemical A&B Chart.

Along with fats, carbohydrates are main suppliers of energy and rich in necessary fiber. We need to eat carbohydrates. However, in order to do what's best for our bodies, it's important to distinguish between three groups of carbohydrates: Group I, II, and III.

GROUP I—Yellow on the A&B Chart

These are the base-building carbohydrates. They may be eaten in unlimited amounts as long as you abide by the A&B principles.

GROUP II—White on the A&B Chart

These natural, but processed carbohydrates may be eaten daily but, to play it safe, they should be eaten with base-builders such as vegetables, salads, and compatible "A" fruits.

These are the unhealthy carbohydrates. Although they are NEVER as unhealthy as bad and extremely-bad proteins whose toxic debris is VERY harmful. Whatever fairytale you have been told…chocolate, eaten compatibly, is never as unhealthy as a sausage on a bun or hamburger on a roll!

Essential #4
When It Comes to Carbohydrates
Chew, Chew, Chew

As you know, saliva is needed for the first step in carbohydrate digestion because it contains amylase, whose primary function is to split the starches (complex carbohydrates) and compound sugars (disaccharides) into smaller units or simple sugars.

The more you chew, the easier it is for your body to properly digest carbohydrates. Chewing is vital to properly digesting carbohydrates; according to the latest research, ideally 25 to 40 times per bite.

Essential #5
Enhance Liver Function
with the Right Eating Schedule

The liver is responsible for regulating so many bodily functions that it is often referred to as "the custodian of the interior milieu." One of the liver's most important jobs is to remove damaged cells and toxins from the blood.

Yes, it is your liver that works hard to get rid of the poison created by your daily metabolism. And like you, it doesn't want to be bothered while working hard. Therefore, support your liver! *How?* The liver has a natural rhythm; choosing the right time of day to eat certain foods will enhance its efficiency and function. Scientists refer to this as the biological liver rhythm. The biological liver rhythm is based on extensive research conducted by Swedish researcher Eric Abraham Forsgren.[23]

In order to maximize on this natural rhythm, follow the BioChemical A&B Method and consume:

- Base-builders in the morning; such as Milk and Apple Breakfast (or substitute milk with yogurt sweetened with artificial sweetener), or other "B" fruits; or in the very least, just fruit if you don't like milk or yogurt.
- Healthy, good proteins: salads, vegetables, and fruits from the "Neutral" or "B" group at midday.
- Carbohydrates from the "A" group along with "Neutral" foods in the afternoon and evening.

Essential #6:
Breathing Correctly is as Important as Eating and Drinking

Correct breathing has far more impact on our health than generally known. Deep breathing exercises massage the abdominal region, which in turn improves both blood circulation and the lymphatic system. This aids your metabolism and thereby the metabolism of fat. If you walk or workout on a regular basis you already benefit from deep breathing.

For the inactive crowd, set aside a few moments each day to take 100 deep, deep breaths. Lie down and take in slow, deep breaths; first breathing in to expand and fill your lungs; then letting it out very slowly and rhythmically. Aside from improving your blood and lymphatic system, you will feel greatly refreshed. A good investment of 5-10 minutes!

Essential #7:
Focus on Chemistry; Not Counting Calories

The BioChemical A&B Method is NOT A DIET, so throw the calorie counter and glycemic index charts out the window. Diets are a temporary measure—no one stays on a diet forever, right?

The BioChemical A&B Method is about knowledge. Knowing how your body works and how the fuel you put into your BioChemical Machine makes it run will serve you for the rest of your life. As long as you eat foods that are chemically compatible with your body chemistry your body will respond by naturally returning to its ideal state: the perfect weight, full of energy, and pain free.

The BIG SEVEN ESSENTIALS

1. You can eat "Neutrals" 24 hours a day; 7 days a week. Eat from Group "A"—Eat from Group "B," But **AVOID** eating **both** at the same meal.

2. Replace bad proteins with good proteins.

3. Eat more of the right foods: base-builders, good proteins, and healthy carbohydrates.

4. When it comes to carbohydrates: Chew, Chew, Chew.

5. Enhance liver function with the right eating schedule.

6. Breathing correctly is as important as eating and drinking.

7. Focus on chemistry; no counting calories or glycemic indexes.

Chapter 6

SOME IMPORTANT SPECIFICS
About Losing Weight—and Keeping the Perfect Weight Forever

The BioChemical A&B Method is NOT a diet. If you follow this method you will never be hungry while in the process of losing weight. Weight loss is just a side effect of balancing your body chemistry. With the A&B Method you don't need to torture yourself through a strict regimen and you don't have to be a part of the 90% of dieters who lapse back into their old ways. Remember the "Yo-Yo" effect? The more diets you try… the less likely you will lose weight.

The BioChemical A&B Method is a permanent lifestyle adjustment that is easy to follow and very healthy. However, as is true with any change to your lifestyle, there are some specifics that you need to know to keep on track:

- The more you weigh when you start the BioChemical A&B Method, the faster you'll shed pounds.

- After your initial success your weight will plateau—it will seem like you're stuck...at least on the scale. Don't be fooled. Your body is in the process of returning to its natural state of chemical balance. Just keep following the BioChemical A&B Method.

- During this time, as your body works hard to get rid of toxins, don't eat chemically incompatible food (yes, I'm talking about a Big Mac). Allow your body to cleanse itself for at least six weeks to balance its chemistry and get rid of the poisons...*before* giving into temptations.

- Don't be concerned if the initial weight-loss isn't concentrated on the bodily areas you would like it to be. If you stick to the BioChemical A&B Method you will eventually lose weight all over your body: face, hands, abdomen, thighs, and legs.

- Don't stress. It takes time for your body to get rid of its poison and for your weight to return to its ideal state. Avoid weighing yourself everyday. Do the "jeans test"* instead. As you regain your good heath you will experience phases that will not be evident on a scale.

- Moderate jogging, a brisk, or ½ hour "normal" walk each day will encourage blood circulation; support the work of your BioChemical Machine; and accelerate the process of getting rid of superfluous pounds—forever. Strenuous sport-walking is not essential with the BioChemical A&B Method.

(Fun!) BioChemical Machine Fact: "The Jeans Test". After approximately six weeks of following the BioChemical A&B Method, try slipping on an old pair of jeans that no longer fit. They may still be a bit tight, but you will find that you may be able to close the zipper, or at least get them over your thighs—an exciting milestone on the road to losing weight.

There are variables to how quickly you will shed excess pounds: your age, personal constitution, and level of activity. If under age 35; 20 to 25 pounds in six weeks is not impossible. But I urge you to take your time as you follow the BioChemical A&B Method...*especially in the beginning.*

Later, when you have detoxified your body, your acid-alkaline balance is restored, and you have lost the weight you wanted to lose...it's possible, even likely, that you'll backslide into your old, bad eating habits. *Don't worry if that happens!* Enjoy your hamburger on a bun with fries and a milkshake. Just make sure that your next meal consists of milk and apples, fruits and/or fresh vegetables, and/or salads. A detoxified body can easily deal with a chemically incompatible meal as long as you bolster its alkaline reserve by returning to the BioChemical A&B Method.

An Apple (or more) a Day

Remember the old saying? Well—apples with whole milk or yogurt can take the stress out of losing weight— plus they're tasty and healthy.

- Begin your day with a breakfast of whole milk and apples. You won't be hungry for 4–5 hours and you'll have a great foundation for the day—or substitute the milk with yogurt sweetened with artificial sweetener and pour over apples cut up into bite-size pieces. Delicious!

- Apples stimulate the metabolism and supply many important phytochemicals.

- The high fiber content of apples helps keep blood sugar levels steady for long periods of time, which naturally curbs the appetite. Eaten with milk they are a great way to detoxify your BioChemical Machine on a daily basis.

Finally, it's important to remember that you might experience an initial *healing process* (healing crisis). For approximately one week you may experience diarrhea, headaches, and shooting pains. This adjustment can differ based on age or current state of health. Don't worry—this will pass after approximately one week. What you may be experiencing is a "shock to the system" as your body begins the hard work of ridding itself of toxins. The good news is that this process is the first step towards getting rid of unwanted pounds as well as poisons.

PART III

DANGEROUS MISCONCEPTIONS

Chapter 7

Big FAT Myths:
The Important Role of Fat

As stated earlier, the myth that "fat makes fat" is at best untrue; at worst potentially dangerous. It also happens to be one of the diet industry's best moneymaking ideas.

In fact fat is the body's number one energy supplier making it very important to our overall health. Fats, oils, fat-containing foods, and yes, even saturated fats play an important role in nourishing our BioChemical Machine. It stores energy, insulates body tissues, and transports fat-soluble vitamins to the blood, as well as plays a key role in cell structure and hormone production. Fat helps develop healthy bones and protects our organs from harm.

BioChemical Machine Fact: Fats can reduce high cholesterol. The body needs fat to function properly.

Yet "fat makes fat" has been hammered into our minds, until we finally accepted the idea of our bodies being a sort of bacon-rind, a combination of lean meat with excess fat that must be eliminated by burning it off. Gurus will have you believe that a simple exercise session or two each and every day will burn away the fat by burning calories and solve all your health and weight problems.

It sounds like a logical association: fry a piece of bacon and it becomes liquid fat—fat that can be poured off. That's how we came to imagine our bodies to work. Exercise, sweat, and the fat will burn and burn and burn so that it will somehow disappear, right? But this is not the case.

As we have seen, according to their chemistry, fats and oils belong to the "Neutral" group. They do not require special treatment to prepare them for digestion in the small intestine.[24]

If you follow the A&B principles...healthy fat will not *make* you fat. The truth is that a total of 60 to 80 grams (3–4 ounces) of healthy fats and oils is the correct daily amount for a healthy, moderately active person. Try to figure out how much you can eat over the course of a day to reach a total of 3 to 4 ounces of fat. You will be surprised.*

---

*If you have already developed a disease, you should discuss the quantity of fats and oils with your doctor.

However, there is a vast difference between healthy and unhealthy fats. The trick is knowing the difference.

UNHEALTHY FATS:

Industrialized fats, especially trans fat (trans fatty acid), whether they are saturated or unsaturated, are unhealthy fats. Trans fatty acids are naturally found in foods like milk in small amounts (2-4%), but particularly produced by heating fats (some margarines contain up to 25%). Trans fat is a human made substance (generally used by restaurants to fry chicken, French fries, etc. because it's cheap). Trans fatty acids disrupt cellular functioning.

HEALTHY FATS:

Healthy fats are natural, cold-pressed oils or virgin oils (no heat or chemicals). Since these oils aren't subjected to the refining process, they are rich in vitamins and essential acids. All natural, unsaturated oils are rich in the essential fatty acids vital to your body's ability to carry out important functions. Of all vegetable oils, linseed (flaxseed) and olive oil are the healthiest.

BioChemical Machine Fact: Research suggests that olive oil is especially beneficial when it comes to the heart. Olive oil protects against heart disease by acting as an anticoagulant that thins the blood and cuts the chance of blood clots or stroke-threatening blockages from forming.[25] It also lowers blood pressure. Research at the University of Texas Health Science Center reported that olive oil lowered dangerous LDL* cholesterol by 21 percent in middle-aged men. At the same time, it preserved good HDL** cholesterol levels.[25]

---

*LDL=Low Density Lipoprotein
**HDL=High Density Lipoprotein

Fat Free or Low-Fat Products

Whatever the reason, a misguided attitude about fat has led most people to believe that "fat-free" or "low-fat" products are the solution to their health and weight problems.

But buying into the fat-free, low-fat myth prevents you from eating healthy fats—an enormous problem. According to a study by the American Heart Association, "...very low fat diets can increase a person's bad cholesterol and rob them of essential nutrients, like iron and calcium." Dr. Linda van Horn, also of the American Heart Association concluded, "Low fat diets can be dangerous, and potentially cause harm."[26]

The AHA is not alone in its assessment. Dr. Nancy Ernst of the National Institutes of Health states: "When you leave the fat at the shelf you left the vitamins and minerals also."[26] What's more, the food industry puts an *enormous* amount of sugar in these low-fat products to make them simulate natural fats and taste better. According to a 1999 CBS News report, *"Thirteen tablespoons* of sugar, corn syrup are added to low-fat yogurt."

Meddling with food chemistry doesn't stop there. Processing "Neutral" cream cheeses, sour cream, yogurt, and curd, (such as cottage cheese), into low-fat/nonfat/fat-free products turns them into *unhealthy* acid-builders—the bad proteins (shaded gray on the BioChemical A&B Chart in the "B" column).

If you follow the A&B principles, you may eat butter and all "Neutral" milk products like cream, sour cream, cheese above 60% fat, cottage cheese, and, *of course*, the very healthy natural olive oil, sunflower oil, soy oil, linseed (flaxseed) oil, and sesame oil. These are the fats and oils that your metabolism needs to function properly.

Margarine or Butter

Many people choose margarine over butter acting on the erroneous assumption that it is the *healthy choice.* I've often heard, "I prefer margarine because it contains unsaturated fat—because it is a vegetable product."

What they often forget is that, in contrast to butter, margarine is an artificial product. "Although a vegetable product and "Neutral", the use of commercial margarine is not recommended," explains Professor Claus Leitzmann, the internationally renowned researcher.[27] "The heating process breaks hydrogen bonds creating a product that causes rancidity and hardening in the tissues. Soy margarine is a slightly improved substance, but it is still not recommended in any large quantity." In addition, trans fatty acids are formed when vegetable oils are processed into margarine.[28] No question about it: butter is a base-builder; thus recommended over margarine.

Saturated Fat

Another myth, I'm sure you've heard, is about the evils of saturated fat. Yet if you carefully examine the foods that contain saturated fatty acids—meat and poultry, whole or reduced-fat milk, butter and some vegetable oils like coconut, palm kernel oil, and palm oil[28]—you'll see that something is drastically wrong with the saturated fat hysteria. Butter, coconuts, and whole milk are strong base-builders, as healthy as it gets! Animal fat is not the villain. Rather, it is the COOKED meat and the LACK of healthy fat in reduced-fat milks and cheeses that causes the harm; not butter and whole milk, which are healthy base-builders.

Common misconceptions about nuts provide another example of how false ideas become generally accepted. Nuts are known to be very high in fat content, no question about it, yet they play a role in fat breakdown.

Another example is the often-vilified pizza. Even when its dough is made from refined white flour,* if its topping consists of ingredients from the "Neutral" column—like mushrooms, olives, onions, peppers, and mozzarella (or other cheese above 60% fat)—pizza remains a compatible meal. Only when you add tomato sauce (made from cooked tomatoes), cooked sausages, and pasta sauces with meat from the "B" column do you violate the laws of your body chemistry. The popular white A&B Pizza without cooked tomato sauce is your best choice!

The truth about fat is not as simple as the myth that has been created around it. I often read baffling advice about fat from diet gurus. For example, one guru asserts that "fat retards the digestion of protein," so it should be eaten with carbohydrates. Another diet guru demands exactly the opposite: "only proteins should be combined with fat."

Why would fat retard digestion? Fats and oils do not require any treatment to prepare them for digestion by the small intestine.[29]

---

*People with health problems—LEVEL TWO—are strongly advised to eat a pizza made of whole wheat dough.

Of course, you can baste your Thanksgiving turkey with butter and, of course, you can pour butter with herbs over your fish fillet. You can even indulge in bacon and eggs (yolks only) if you wish. And, of course, you can eat whole wheat bread with mayonnaise, tomatoes, and onions—or baked potatoes with butter, dill, salt and pepper. And, there is nothing wrong with eating natural rice with fried onions; spaghetti with butter, mushrooms, cream, and peas; or banana flambé. The issue is to maintain the acid-alkaline balance by carefully following the BioChemical A&B Chart.

Fat doesn't make you fat; rather, the *lack* of fat deprives you of important vitamins and minerals and can contribute to cell degeneration and illness. Your metabolism will function perfectly if you choose the right foods as outlined by the BioChemical A&B Method. If you have reached the age when cells slow down and/or have developed a chronic disease then abide by the LEVEL TWO chart which emphasizes 80% base-builders and 20% **healthy** acid-builders and avoid the bad and extremely-bad proteins.

Otherwise, you can dispense with the myths you've heard about fat. Understanding the match between food chemistry and body chemistry ensures that you know more than the diet gurus. That's how you will stay slim, energetic, healthy, and happy.

Chapter 8

THE TRUTH ABOUT CHOLESTEROL
And What You Don't Know About Homocysteine

It seems like every time we hear about cholesterol and saturated fat, it's linked to some ad promoting the latest and greatest "magic pill." In an interview on ABC's 20/20, Dr. Thomas James, president of the American Heart Association, (at the time of the interview) stated that a single anti-cholesterol drug released that year from one of the major pharmaceutical manufacturers generated *"a three billion dollar positive cash flow."*[30]

Cholesterol has become big business. But is it true that it's as big a nutritional devil as we've been led to believe? And is it true that saturated fat is responsible for dangerously high cholesterol in the blood? Not entirely.

111

As is true with fat, there are many misconceptions about cholesterol. The fact is that cholesterol is vital for the immune system and nearly all body cells. It is an integral part of all cell membranes and is a required component for building cell walls. It is the starting point for the production of steroid hormones, including the sex hormones. And you may be surprised to learn that cholesterol—once it is broken down by the liver into bile salts—helps your body decompose fat.[31] Two-thirds of your body's cholesterol is produced in your own liver.* The rest comes from the foods we eat.

But not all cholesterol is the same. There are two different kinds that function in your body.

HDL: The Good Cholesterol

Cholesterol is an essential component of lipoproteins, which transport fats and fatty acids in the bloodstream to tissue throughout the body. High-density lipoprotein (HDL) cholesterol acts as a scavenger, transporting fat and cholesterol from these tissues to the liver. Most of the cholesterol in the blood is in the form of high-density lipoproteins that helps us protect against arterial disease. HDL picks up cholesterol in the arteries and takes it back to the liver for excretion or reprocessing. HDL is often referred to as "good cholesterol."

---

*The liver has many regulatory and storage functions. It receives the products of digestion, converts glucose to glycogen (as long-chain carbohydrates used for storage), and breaks down fats. It removes excess amino acids from the blood, converting them to urea, which is excreted by the kidneys. The liver also produces bile and blood-clotting factors, and removes damaged red cells and toxins, such as alcohol, from the blood.—*Time* (November 24, 1997, page 83) reported in the Health sector that "a landmark study" has shown that vegetarians had higher blood levels of lipoprotein "a." Furthermore, "a new analysis by a joint US-Italian team shows...that the fish eaters have an average 40% lower level of this particular lipoprotein."

LDL: What You Don't Know About Bad Cholesterol

You're probably already familiar with low-density lipoprotein (LDL), the so-called "bad cholesterol." According to conventional wisdom, saturated fat in the diet increases the LDL, which in turn increases the risk of heart disease. While it is true that LDL, in excess, can become deposited on the surface of the arteries, which in turn can lead to arteriosclerosis; it is not true that this can be avoided simply by omitting saturated fat from your diet.

Even if unsaturated fat-acids lower the cholesterol in the blood, it does not mean that omitting saturated fats makes everything all right. The truth is that your body can easily process saturated fat, just as it can process your own production of cholesterol...as long as your metabolism is functioning as it should.

All body functions are interrelated like stones in a mosaic. Take away one stone and the picture becomes less than perfect. Eliminating saturated fat from your diet is *not* the answer to lowering high cholesterol. In fact doing so may affect your body chemistry adversely in other ways.

- Recent studies at the University of California at Los Angeles (UCLA) were conducted in which cholesterol levels in the blood were reduced by retaining it in the intestine (and interrupting its absorption into the bloodstream). Yet doing so resulted in only 1.8% fewer heart attacks—while the incidence of cancer increased by 5%.

Homocysteine: Another Stone in the Mosaic

In the big picture of your health, it's not only LDL cholesterol that can damage arteries and lead to heart attacks and stroke. An amino acid called homocysteine can also play a part. High homocysteine levels in the blood can cause cholesterol to change to something called oxidized low-density lipoprotein, which is more damaging to the arteries than LDL. In addition, high homocysteine levels can make blood clot more easily than it should; increasing the risk of blood vessel blockages. A blockage can cause strokes or interrupt blood flow. Up to 20% of people with heart disease have high homocysteine levels.

According to Dr. Kilian Robinson of the Cleveland Clinic, "You can have normal cholesterol and normal blood pressure—but high homocysteine is often the only detectable reason why you might experience a vascular episode, heart attack or stroke."[30] He added, "High homocysteine may be just as important and widespread as a cardiac factor." Homocysteine is produced by eating extremely-bad proteins, like cooked meat and bad proteins, such as cooked fish and cheese below 50% fat. Deficiencies of vitamin B also cause homocysteine to build up in the body.

Dr. Kilmer McCully, a pathologist at Harvard University and Massachusetts Hospital, linked homocysteine to vitamin B deficiency...30 years ago![30] But his research was ignored. Instead, federal money was poured into cholesterol research.

Dr. Thomas James, former president of the American Heart Association said, "Pharmaceutical companies didn't want to fund homocysteine research because there was no money in the cure."[30] Most people with a high homocysteine level don't get enough folate (also called folic acid), vitamin B_6, or vitamin B_{12} in their diet. Replacing these vitamins by eating the right foods helps return the homocysteine level to normal.

Your body is a finely tuned BioChemical machine. Keeping its complex chemical make-up balanced is the key to good health—not omitting certain foods from your diet...even those that contain saturated fat. If you always ate according to the perfect match of food chemistry and body chemistry, you would not build up bad cholesterol or homocysteine.

Plainly put, you need to increase the intake of base-builders instead of lowering or omitting saturated fats. If you have already developed chronic diseases, you should avoid every food item that is marked by the color gray and red on the LEVEL TWO A&B Chart. However, you may eat all "Neutral" products including butter, smoked fish, cured meat or rolled ham, salami, sour cream, cheese *above* 60% fat and many other food items. These are all products containing saturated fat— supposedly responsible for the increase in cholesterol and risk of heart disease, which is not the case.

If you have high cholesterol, you should place special emphasis on whole wheat products while avoiding *unhealthy* acid-builders such as white flour or white rice and balancing your diet between 80% base-builders *(yellow)* and 20% (healthy) acid-builders *(white)*.

The unsaturated fat-acids and rich fibers like cellulose and hemicellulose in these foods lower the cholesterol in the blood and fiber binds cholesterol.

Also, you should studiously avoid trans fat, the unnatural and highly processed fat that is cheaply manufactured for use in restaurants to fry things like French fries.

After four weeks, your cholesterol will be significantly reduced; blood circulation will improve and the risk of arteriosclerosis will be minimized. These are all just some of side benefits of following the A&B principles.

Chapter 9

TRUE OR FALSE
Can Tofu Fight Cancer?

If your doctor tells you that you have cancer, you feel as if a jury has convicted you of a crime you didn't commit. Because of its insidious nature, cancer is not an illness that can be treated with a 100% predictable outcome. I remember how devastated I was when I found out that I had cancer and would be losing my kidneys. I know how it feels to be desperately looking for something that can save your life. Reaching for every hope; every straw; every illusion is better than just helplessly looking forward to becoming sicker and sicker—until the day you die.

So I can truly understand how a simple food item, such as tofu, could be set up as having almost magical anti-cancer properties. "Like other beans, soybeans contain the anti-cancer compounds protease inhibitors," writes the diet-author, Judy Lin Eftekar in her book, *Feed Yourself Right.*[32] "Researchers at Japan's National Cancer Center noted that people who eat macrobiotic miso soup every day (a popular soup made from soybean paste) are 33% less likely to have stomach cancer...Substituting meat with soy products like tofu or texturized vegetable protein (TVP) has been shown to reduce the risk of breast cancer..."

Studies may seem to indicate that soy reduces the risk of cancer, but how can anyone know for certain? Statistics are not proof of cause and effect. Gurus have twisted the research about tofu to present it in a way that is misleading to people desperate to pin their hopes on something that might help them in their darkest hour.

This is not to say that tofu and its potential to deter cancer should be ignored. In the course of my research, I asked the renowned authority, Professor Claus Leitzmann to elaborate about tofu's beneficial qualities. "Tofu contains, besides many other substances, genistein (phytoestrogen*), which has anti-carcinogenic properties. The protein of the soybean is high-grade. The acid-basic actions are a question of the quantity of consumption."

He also mentioned that "...East Asian people would profit from the consumption of tofu...yet, the isolation and application of the effective substances are problematic."

---

*The phytoestrogens are divided into two groups: the Isaflavonoids and the Lignans. Well-known Isoflavonoids are genistein and daidzein. These are found only in legumes (soybean, etc.) of the tropics. Traditional Asian nourishment consists of a multiple of isoflavonoids by contrast to that of the American and European. As a result, the Asians are far less often afflicted with hormone-dependent conditions such as breast cancer. However, highly processed soybean products, such as soy sauce or tofu, do not contain the high levels of genistein found in unprocessed soybeans. As of this writing, isolation of phytoestrogens, such as genistein, has been unsuccessful. Therefore, equally effective phytoestrogens are not yet available to the consumer market in a supplement form. (Watzl, Bernhard; Leitzmann, Claus: *Bioactive Substances in Food*, Hippokrates Publ., 1999).

Too much emphasis has been bestowed on the diets of Asian men and women and how their consumption of soy products *might* offer a form of cancer prevention. "Might", of course, is an important qualifier; there's no definitive proof. In addition, many tout that if most of your protein comes from "fat-free" soy products you are able to avoid beef and other high-fat meats.

Let's dispense with some of the misconceptions about soy. First of all, it is *not* fat-free. Soybeans contain 20% fat; the highest ratio among legumes. The soybean itself belongs to the legume family that includes beans, peas, and lentils. This means soybeans, rich in good protein, belong to the "Neutral" food group. Do you remember our slogan about "Neutrals" on the A&B Chart: *"24 hours a day, 7 days a week?"*

However, tofu is a *processed* food item made of soymilk containing 5 to 8% protein, 3 to 4% fat, 2 to 4% carbohydrates, and 0.6% minerals. Soymilk is made of soybeans, a healthy, base-building plant. However, in order to produce soymilk, soybeans are soaked for only 12 hours in a 10:1 ratio of water. Beans (EVERY BEAN) need to be soaked in water for many more hours in order to activate the chemical process, which ultimately turns them into a healthy food item. Afterwards, the soaked soybeans are ground and heated to 100 degrees Celsius (212 degrees Fahrenheit) and centrifuged. During this process, the so-called soymilk emerges, from which tofu is made.[33]

The most damaging information I have ever read from spreading and misleading messages about tofu was a book by a diet guru who openly refers to Dr. Hay's research. This guru also speaks of the acid-alkaline balance, yet the book was crowded with mistakes about chemistry. The major problem was that this guru

119

recommended tofu as a base-builder, which is dangerous advice for someone battling a major disease. Base-builders, YELLOW on the BioChemical A&B Chart, can and *should* be eaten as much as possible every day. This is *not* the case with tofu. Unfortunately, many cancer patients believe such advice and cling to the hope that eating huge amounts of tofu can help overcome their disease.

To be honest, if I had cancer and didn't know about the BioChemical A&B Method, I would start eating tofu like crazy too; hoping that it would save me. The fact that Asians are famous for their health might influence me that there was a "wonder antidote" that needed to be eaten. However, this is not the case nor the reason diet gurus are "selling" their miraculous tofu diets to you.

First of all, Asians eat a bit differently than the way described by gurus who have, obviously, discovered that Asian diets and alternative medicines are marketable. Secondly, lumping all Asians into one category is vague since culture and cuisine differs from country to country; from eating habits to eating habits; and from poor to rich. Which Asian population is the basis for tofu's cancer fighting properties—the Chinese, Japanese, Korean, Vietnamese, Tibetan, Philippine, or Taiwanese?

For example, let's take the Chinese...considered by many to be among the healthiest people on earth. Can their high standard of health be attributed to eating huge portions of tofu, miso, and other soy products? It's more likely that their primary diet of vegetables, salads, sprouts (a natural soybean and a strong base-builder), fruits, and rice lends them the properties they need for good health. Additionally, for the Chinese, cooked meat, fish, or (processed) tofu are delicacies—eaten only from time to time in addition to their basic foods.

One of the reasons the Chinese are in such good health is that their traditional eating habits mirror the BioChemical A&B Method, unintentionally matching the chemistry of the foods they eat with their body chemistry.

For example, rice is found in the "A" column; vegetables, salads, and tofu are "Neutral". Chemically, that's the perfect combination. Even the famous Peking duck with oranges or nectarines naturally follows the BioChemical A&B Chart. Meat is a strong acid-builder and "B" fruits are strong base-builders, which neutralize the acid as long as no third-party foods from the "A" column join the digestion process. The truth is that Asian eating patterns are very much like that of our early ancestors.

China is, at this time, a "so-called" developing country. These people are relatively poor; therefore, it is not unusual for a large family to consume meat like chicken, pork, or beef *only on special occasions*.

These habits echo those of our (Western world) ancestors and are still very much the case in other Arabian and African countries where you'll find the oldest and healthiest people on earth. Reaching the age of 100 is not unusual.

Yet, longevity has nothing to do with race. As Professor Claus Leitzmann said, "The Caucasus people can reach the highest ages; over 100 years is common!" He's right. The secret to a long, healthy life lies in making sure the nourishment of our cells are chemically balanced.

Fortunately, in our western world, many progressive medical doctors consider the eating habits of their patients in the recovery treatment of diseases; including cancer. If you are fighting disease, you should abide by the LEVEL TWO A&B Chart. On that chart, you can see that tofu is a perfectly healthy, beneficial food when eaten the A&B way; which is to eat as much from the YELLOW group as possible; moderately of the WHITE group (where you'll find tofu); and rarely, if at all, from the RED & GRAY groups.

Following the BioChemical A&B Method is a vital way to bolster your immune system in its fight against disease. Don't be fooled into thinking one food, like tofu, can single-handedly solve your health problems. A comprehensive dietary program based on the A&B principles will enable your body to dedicate its full resources toward getting better. Later chapters will talk about some of the specific foods you should be eating to optimize your body's ability to heal. If you do so, I believe your body will respond the same as mine did and continues to do.

PART IV

THE
MILK & APPLE
THERAPY

Chapter 10

THE TRUTH ABOUT MILK

The first food we eat when we come into the world is milk. Mother's milk is nature's perfect food. Mostly water; the remainder is made up of 6.9% carbohydrates, 3.7% fat, 1.2% protein, lactose, pantothenic acid, potassium, phosphorus, iron, and vitamins A, B_1, B_2, B_6, D, and C. As infants, incapable of digesting regular food, milk is the ideal food for our developing BioChemical machines. In a sense, infants "eat" milk as it is the only source of their nourishment. As we get older, we no longer "eat" milk. Instead, we drink it. Now, it's no longer human milk, but cow's milk; ideally whole and organic. Due to its processing, milk's composition has shifted to 3.4% protein, 3.4% fat, and 4.7% carbohydrates, but it's still good for us and we consume it with our breakfast, lunch, and dinner because we know it helps our body's calcium requirements.

As everyone knows, milk and milk products are loaded with calcium. What's more, one glass of whole milk (250 ml) contains only 8 grams of fat; a fragment of the total of 60 to 80 grams of fat that may be eaten over the course of a day by healthy, moderately active people. In so many ways milk is, in a word: Great!

- Calcium is important not only for healthy bones, but also for skin, hair, eyesight, cell growth, and thyroid gland functions.

- "A daily under-supply of 300 mg calcium means the loss of 10% bone-mass within one year," according to Professor Helmuth Minne, University of Heidelberg.

- "Without calcium, nerves and muscles cannot function, our heart wouldn't beat regularly, and the blood wouldn't clot" Professor Minne further states. "In order to make calcium accessible to your bones, you need vitamin D, which is also found in milk. Vitamin D is the key which opens the door to bones for calcium to enter."[34]

- A study at the University of California at San Diego showed that people who drank milk were one-third less likely to develop colorectal cancer than those who didn't.[35]

- Another study at the University of California at San Diego showed that acidophilus milk, a fermented form of milk, is a deterrent against colon cancer.[35]

- In another research study, at the University of California at San Diego, milk was linked to a decreased incidence of stomach and lung cancer.

And the calcium in milk may help prevent intestinal cancer.[35]

- Non-milk drinkers are twice as likely to have high blood pressure as those who drink milk... according to a study of 8,000 men by the National Heart, Lung and Blood Institute.

- Through extensive research, scientists at the University of California at San Diego discovered that milk contains an amazing property besides calcium—an "unidentified factor" that has been shown to retard bone disease and control blood pressure.[35]

Despite so many scientifically established benefits, self-appointed diet "experts" have reviled milk and milk products for years. Unfortunately, many have bought into this nonsense. Although, the dairy industry has made the mistake of adding hormones, antibiotics, and chemicals to their products, increasing numbers of dairy farmers are producing hormone-, antibiotic-, and pesticide-free whole milk today. Ask for it! The more people ask—the more organic whole milk will become available.

You may say that you can't drink milk because you're lactose intolerant. Well, you wouldn't be alone. However it's not a condition that should stand in your way of enjoying the benefits of milk.

Lactose Intolerance

"The milk of cows, goats, and sheep is often consumed by humans, but only Western societies drink milk after infancy; for people in most of the world, milk causes flatulence and diarrhea," states *Webster's Encyclopedia.*[36] Two-thirds of the world's population gets sick from drinking milk because they lack the enzyme to digest cow's milk—otherwise known as lactose intolerance.

Why is this so common if milk is so healthy? The answer is in the way we *consume* milk. To do so in a healthy way requires knowledge about matching the food chemistry with the chemistry of the body.

I was captivated with the fact that "only Western societies drink milk after infancy." The Bedouins in Arabia and North Africa and others who retained the eating habits of their ancestors won't *drink* cow, goat, or sheep milk. Instead, milk is processed into yogurt, sour milk, Kefir, and cheese; all of which are good protein "Neutral" food items. Only infants drink milk in these cultures. For adults, goat or camel milk is eaten in the forms described above; usually as a complete meal to which other foods *are not* added.

Here's where the Western world encounters its problem with milk: We usually consume milk with the wrong foods like cereal, bread, potatoes, rice, or pasta. Remember, processed milk products such as yogurt, heavy cream, sour milk, whey, and cream cheese are "Neutral" and can be eaten with cereal, bread, potatoes, rice, pasta and sugar products—but *not* with the liquid form of milk, which if you refer to the BioChemical A&B Chart can be found in the "B" column.

We must understand that homogenizing and pasteurizing interferes with nature. Original whole milk was (before being homogenized and pasteurized) a strong base-builder, belonging to the "Neutrals", therefore easy to digest and very healthy. It could be eaten with anything...including cereal, bread, potatoes, rice, or pasta. But this doesn't apply to the milk we buy in supermarkets today that has been changed through the industrial process. Yet, despite the processing of milk, it remains a moderate base-builder with its healthy vitamins A, D, B_2, B_{12}, H, and minerals intact, as well as the "unidentified factor" that researchers discovered.

So how can we capitalize on the healthy aspects of milk? The answer is simple—"eat" milk with base-forming foods, such as apples, pineapples, oranges, melons, and other exotic fruits from the "B" column—and, of course, "Neutral" foods, especially "Neutral" cheeses. Due to its detoxifying effect on our system, it is an excellent idea to consume whole milk in the morning with other strong base-builders, especially apples, which I'll expound upon in later chapters. Avoid consuming milk with foods from the "A" column like bananas, raisins, grapes, figs, and dates.

BioChemical Machine Fact: *It's very important to keep in mind that you may go through a so-called HEALING PROCESS (an adjustment period) while the body works hard to get rid of the poison.*

For approximately one week you *might* experience diarrhea, headaches, and shooting pains. This adjustment differs based on age or current state of health.

> **BioChemical Machine Fact:** *This HEALING PROCESS can be (and often is) mistaken for LACTOSE INTOLERANCE due to a similarity of symptoms!*

Don't worry. Just stick to the A&B principles; soon, you'll be amazed that you can drink milk without experiencing any discomfort.

> **BioChemical Machine Fact:** *There are some RARE cases of people who suffer from MILK-PROTEIN ALLERGY. They must avoid dairy products or eat them according to their physician's advice.*

The most important calcium suppliers are milk and milk products. Many vegetables and herbs such as parsley, chives, and dill offer a relatively high calcium content; however, the body cannot utilize them as easily as milk and milk products. If you are still reluctant to drink milk, you can still reap its benefits by consuming other dairy products from the "Neutral" group, such as yogurt, buttermilk, whey or Kefir, cream, sour cream, cottage cheese, cream cheese, or goat's milk cheese.

> **BioChemical Machine Fact:** *In addition to the other benefits, YOGURT counteracts bacteria that cause urinary infections.*

The most impressive quality of milk may be the relief it can provide for the 38 million Americans who suffer from arthritis[37] or osteoporosis. I am one of them. For many years, I refused to drink milk because of the chemicals, hormones, antibiotics, and pesticides found in milk.

However, when I became crippled by rheumatoid arthritis, I began following a diet based on 80% base-builders and only 20% *healthy* acid-builders. This change in my eating habits included consuming milk with peaches and oranges. Then, I made a revolutionary discovery—a story I will share with you in the next chapter.

Chapter 11

ARTHRITIS & A TRUE
MIRACLE DRUG

Unfortunately, we often fail to follow good advice until it's too late. And so it was with my milk consumption. Put off by its chemicals and hormones, I avoided drinking milk every day. For fifteen years, I followed the basic A&B principles and felt great.

I overlooked the fact that by age thirty cell activity begins to slow down; a decline that only accelerates as we get older. I just felt *too* good. I didn't consider taking preventive steps to address this change; namely eating 80% base-builders and only 20% acid-builders as was recommended in Dr. Hay's original work. (I had not yet discovered the vast difference between healthy and unhealthy acid-builders.) I also wasn't avoiding bad and extremely-bad proteins as one should; especially after surgery. Instead, I indulged in an excess of bad and extremely-bad proteins. Why would I take such a chance with my health? I didn't know any better! *Because my most important discovery had not yet been made!* That would come much later.

Further developing Dr. Hay's work and supported by encouragement from the Chairman of the Department of Chemistry at Rutgers University, Professor Luke Burke, I would soon have the solution. I was on the verge of making my most important discovery: that two different types of digestion exist for protein, and the vast chemical difference between "good" and "bad" proteins. These revolutionary findings would ultimately lead to the development of the BioChemical A&B Chart.

As I look back now, I realize that it was a personal crisis that forced me to dig deeper into Dr. Hay's research—looking for answers in his work for an affliction that was making my life a living hell... arthritis. At that time, I didn't know that lurking around the corner was an ailment that could make life miserable. I never wondered about brittle bones or a crippled body. In my mind, arthritis was something for "old people"—certainly not for me, although I was no longer what we call young. In those days I felt even better and more energetic than when I was in my 20s. Being in great shape, I never imagined that a terrible disease would attack my bones.

Yet, one day pains gradually began in my left thumb. I ignored the pain. I wanted to believe that it was an injury; perhaps caused while training our frisky dog. Soon after, I began to experience increasing pain in my spine, but again, I dismissed it as probably the result of an old riding accident. Over the following months the pain in my thumb increased and after a while I couldn't even hold a cup anymore. The pain started to keep me awake at nights. After a couple of months my thumb became crooked. I was shocked and I tried to straighten it by using force.

After the suffering spread to my feet, legs, knees, hips, and shoulders I finally went to a doctor who told me I had rheumatoid arthritis. He could do no more for me than prescribe painkillers and calcium, which did little to alleviate my pain. Gradually, the agony worsened to the point that I could no longer get up without the help of a cane.

I panicked. But being a researcher, I quickly realized my energy was better spent collecting information. In the course of my research, I kept coming back to the fact that milk can cure some bone problems and possesses the ability to detoxify the body. I guess it was out of desperation that I remembered Hay's teachings about the acid-alkaline balance/reserve and the vital ratio of 80% base-builders and 20% healthy acid-builders. But as I said, at that time I didn't know there was a vast difference between the healthy acid-builders and the unhealthy ones! Or rather, those that you can now find shaded WHITE on the LEVEL TWO of the BioChemical A&B Chart (the healthy acid-builders) and those that are really bad—the GRAY and the RED groups.

The next morning I drank three glasses of whole milk and ate peaches. Of course, I didn't drink low fat or fat-free milk as I knew the dairy industry puts sugar and chemicals into those products to make them taste better and more like whole milk. I took the whole milk like medicine. But my unprepared body reacted adversely to the milk, as if I had consumed camel's milk or castor oil. I called my reaction "races to the bathroom."

I didn't know it at the time, but would later discover that my body's reaction to the milk was a healing process—a normal, temporary period of adjustment in which the body's chemistry corrects and cleanses itself. Later, as I began to test my theories on others, both my personal "guinea pigs" and later on test participants at a private clinic, I discovered that *people were confusing this healing process with "lactose intolerance."* From then on I started my day with whole milk and foods that strictly adhered to the 80% base-builders and not more than 20% acid-builders rule. But the pain didn't really go away.

At that time I lived in a beautiful farm area in New Jersey that was ideal for a researcher. The only things that could interrupt my thinking process were raccoons and rabbits. Since they didn't bother me (instead, my beloved dogs bothered them), I was focused on my increasing and frightening pain.

It was pure chance that my neighbor, the owner of an apple farm, visited me one evening and brought a huge bag of big green Granny Smith apples as a gift. It was also pure chance that the next morning I ate two of these apples together with my "medicine"; the milk. *Why?* I hadn't shopped for a week and my refrigerator was almost empty. There wasn't anything available except milk and apples.

I was surprised to discover that after drinking only one glass of milk (250 ml) and eating two apples, I felt like I had eaten a big, satisfying breakfast! The hunger that usually plagued me by mid-morning never materialized.

Furthermore, by the next day I realized that my pain had lessened! I showed my husband my previously bandaged and stiff thumb, which was now mobile.

Gradually the pain vanished throughout my body. After two weeks of this new "cure" my thumb was flexible. Of course, I was thrilled and completely dedicated to sticking to this new powerhouse union of apples and milk. In the course of my recovery, I became curious. I wanted to uncover the reason behind this amazing discovery.

I knew that the main supplier for energy, besides carbohydrates, is (healthy) fat. For years I had primarily eaten olive oil and butter. But I wanted to find out whether or not the "fat-free," "low-fat" and "2 % fat" milk, combined with apples, would have the same effect as the whole milk. It didn't work. Soon after breakfast, I was very hungry and even felt mild pain in some parts of my body. The reaction of my body was only logical since sugar and chemicals (added to low or no-fat milk by manufacturers for better taste) are unhealthy acid-builders. Besides that, I violated the A&B principles. Apples belong to the food in the "B" column and sugar to the "A" column. Still, I was very surprised by my body's, almost immediate, reaction.

It really hit me when focusing on the fact that I was not hungry for many hours after drinking whole milk and eating the apples in the morning. I was totally fascinated by these results. *What was it that was so powerful?* After a couple of days and a lot of pondering, I realized: *two powerful base-builders were joining forces.* That means your metabolism gets it all: pure vitamins and minerals.

These discoveries captured my scholarly heart. I couldn't resist asking my mother to be my "guinea pig" since she suffered from both lactose intolerance and osteoporosis. She, as many others, grew up with old-fashioned and erroneous ideas about eating. I was convinced that she might have developed lactose intolerance over the course of several decades, especially since she didn't have this problem when I was a child. I wondered if, perhaps, self-poisoning was responsible for the disappearance of the appropriate enzyme required to digest milk? I wanted to determine whether or not my mother could detoxify her body with the A&B principles as I had done. If so, she could start drinking milk, which would help her osteoporosis without experiencing the nasty side-effects of lactose intolerance.

My mother followed the A&B teachings and ate precisely the foods that her body needed. She ate moderate quantities of "Neutral" dairy products or whole milk with apples or other "B" fruits, salads and/or vegetables. One of the first things she reported was that she enjoyed drinking milk for the first time in years—especially with apples. The unpleasant mucous build-up she had always associated with milk disappeared. She also reported feeling more rejuvenated than she had in a long time. Significantly, we discovered that it was NOT the milk alone that caused her lactose intolerance. Once her body chemistry was balanced she could cope with milk again and there were no more symptoms of lactose intolerance.

Her skeleton now benefits from the high calcium content of the whole milk. And the pain she felt from osteoporosis, which has stopped progressing, went away completely.

Two-thirds of the populations in western countries are lactose intolerant. If the Milk & Apple Therapy can have the same impact on others that it had on my mother, then these findings are significant. It would demonstrate that lactose intolerance is, in most cases, nothing but the so-called healing process.

I couldn't resist recruiting friends to participate in my experiment. The result was overwhelming. Everybody who followed the Milk and Apple Therapy and the BioChemical A&B Method was soon able to drink and enjoy whole milk. One of my test subjects wrote the following enthusiastic letter to me on August 19, 1998:

"...By the way, the new eating plan that you gave us is not only easy to follow, but it has also given us a lot more energy! In addition to this, I might add, that we have begun to eat an apple with a glass of milk at the start of each day...like you had suggested. I thought you might also like to know that prior to this, I was unable to drink whole milk, as I was lactose intolerant. However, when I drink the whole milk while eating the apple, I have no negative reactions. I feel healthy and I believe you are right about the cleansing benefits the two of these foods have for the body when eaten together."

As I said, these are not the only cases in the world that testify to the effectiveness of the A&B principles. There arc millions of people in Arabia and Africa who still follow our species' original eating habits. They do not suffer from lactose intolerance, arthritis, and osteoporosis.

But, interestingly enough, wealthy people in Arabia and Africa suffer from the same diseases as we do; no doubt because they have adapted to our Western eating habits.

Only two years after having discovered the Milk & Apple Therapy, I had forgotten the unbearable pain caused by arthritis. I asked myself, "What would happen if I returned to my old eating habits?" I became curious. My scholarly heart was challenged and I couldn't resist trying "the old way". I stopped drinking whole milk and eating apples in the morning. I ate small amounts of potatoes, raw vegetables, salads, and fruits and increased the amount of cooked meat I consumed. I also ate packaged snack foods: cheese curls, barbecued potato chips, and other junk foods.

After a short period of time, mild pain in my hands, joints, and hips began to bother me. I was extremely tired. I experienced increasing pain in my left kidney. After five weeks the pain in my bones, especially the hip, increased dramatically. I needed the help of a cane to get up from the couch and walk. I did what I hadn't done in years; I took heavy painkillers. But the pain didn't stop. My hips and spine ached as badly as they had after a serious riding accident I experienced long ago.

I didn't wait long before I went, in tremendous pain and almost in tears, to a nearby supermarket to buy all kinds of food that increases the body's alkalinity: cauliflower, broccoli, carrots, spinach, white and red cabbage, sprouts, onions, parsley, chives, all kinds of lettuce—and a lot of potatoes. I prepared a huge bowl of salad consisting of lettuce and vegetables, olive oil, apple vinegar, sea salt, and steamed potatoes with skins. I anxiously temporized the waiting period of three hours in order to drink my "medicine" (late in the night): three glasses of whole milk (each glass 250 ml) and two apples. Soon the pain lessened and within a couple of days I was almost back on track. After two weeks I was completely pain-free.

I intentionally repeated this self-experiment four more times. After a period of feeling well, fit and healthy, I would dabble with eating the "old way." Every time the results were the same: pain, lack of energy, and more pain. After four times I decided to leave the clinical tests to clinical researchers and their subjects. I had the proof I needed. Now I knew that this experiment could be done with every person under clinical scientific supervision. Ultimately, the accuracy of my findings was confirmed.

After having personally experienced such overwhelming results, there was no doubt in my mind that whole milk and apples are a true miracle drug. From then on, I tried to convince everyone who was experiencing pain to convert their eating habits to the BioChemical A&B Method and at least give the Milk & Apple Therapy a try.

Despite my good intentions, I often faced tremendous skepticism. "Try it at least for a couple of days" I would urge, "You have nothing to lose and so much to gain!" Only those who were already seriously ill and full of pain followed my advice. I managed to convince my husband—a true skeptic. When the pain of his arthritis became so bad that he could hardly climb the stairs in our house, he decided it couldn't hurt to try the A&B Method and Milk & Apple Therapy.

After a short period of time, he experienced the same results as everyone else and cured his arthritis. Others found a breakfast consisting of milk and apples...simply bizarre. "Why would this have such a profound effect on my well-being?" was the most common question I heard. I never got tired of explaining the reason behind the Milk & Apple Therapy's effectiveness: *Two base-builders join forces.* Apples, a strong base-builder, support the unique effects of milk, which even in its treated (pasteurized) form remains a moderate base-builder.

And I referred again and again to the scientific studies conducted at the University of California at San Diego supporting the *unidentified factor in milk* that is so beneficial to our health.

I pondered to myself: "What exactly is the secret behind milk and apples?" I found the answer from studying the example of a baby. If a baby vomits mother's milk, the milk comes out already "curdled" by the stomach's acidity. The same is true for milk products that have been made sour. This curdling is a fermentation process caused through enzymatic lactic acid that prepares food for digestion.

This example opened my eyes to the logic behind Milk and Apple Therapy's success: "B" fruits are not only strong base-builders, but also contain fruit-acid (a short-term acid supply). In short, milk and "B" fruits are a symbiosis that promotes the digestion. The simultaneous delivery of alkalinity by two powerful base-builders—and the effectiveness with which it can detoxify the body is the reason why milk and apples could cure my arthritis, my mother's lactose intolerance, and my husband's arthritis. We all swear by this true miracle therapy and wouldn't change our breakfast for anything in this world.

I was determined to convince people that this approach to food was the smart way to balance out our interference with nature. One of those whom I converted to my cause was a 55-year-old American worker. On May 25, 1998, after only two weeks of following the BioChemical A&B Method, he wrote the following letter:

"In 1991, I was working as a warehouse person in New Jersey. While unloading a truck of padding for wall-to-wall carpet, I twisted my back, causing me to leave work for almost two weeks.

When I returned to work, my back was never the same. I eventually left work and applied for workers compensation... In August of 1994 I was diagnosed with osteo-arthritis. I saw doctors at Metropolitan Hospital's Orthopedic Department in New York City and also spoke with Orthopedic Surgeons at Albany Medical Center, Albany, New York. The diagnosis was firm...I couldn't work, run, lift heavy objects, climb stairs without effort, or play with my children. I was placed on anti-inflammatory drugs (non-steroidal) and pain medication was prescribed. I was told not to do anything high impact that could cause further injury to my hips.

In May of 1998, I had the good fortune of meeting Eleonora De Lennart through my wife. De Lennart learned that I had osteoarthritis and asked to meet me. With reluctance I went to her home and spoke with her. She asked me all kinds of questions.

All I thought of was 'how much is this consultation going to cost?' She told me that she also was arthritic to the point that [she had] some deformity in her fingers. I said to myself 'Yeah, right'. De Lennart told me that if I changed my eating habits I could possibly go back to a normal life.... Although I've just started trying what she has advised, the results are amazing. I have a low tolerance for milk, so using plain yogurt and apples, I decided to give it a try. On Monday, May 11, 1998, I started my day with two eight (8) ounce glasses of blended plain yogurt and two delicious apples.

I felt like I had eaten a whole breakfast, which I never do. I had to sit down and relax because I was so full.

After following her recommendations, about eight days later I had a burst of energy and decided to try to work in the yard raking leaves and pruning some trees and bushes. I put in about five hours of yard work which I haven't done in the past four years. The thing I noticed

143

most was I didn't seem to have a need for my pain medication which I usually take after any physical exertion. I still took my anti-inflammatory. The daily pain I had been experiencing decreased a lot. I also made mention to my wife that I felt pretty good after doing that work. I don't know what the process is, but I do know that I'm not walking with much of a gait anymore, I can walk up stairs with less effort, and the range of motion concerning my hips has greatly improved. I know different things work for different people, but I firmly believe that meeting Eleonora De Lennart has changed my life.

She's shown me how to change my eating habits and because of this, though I'm not 100%, I'm 65% and getting better..."

Since that first letter, he exchanged the yogurt with milk and is recovering dramatically. Recently he paid me a visit. He literally came dancing into my house, shouting, "I love you! I love you! You changed my life!"

You may question the dramatic results of following the BioChemical A&B Method, but EVERYBODY in my experimentation has had similar results. Even if you're a skeptic...you have nothing to lose by at least trying the BioChemical A&B Method—especially if you're suffering from pain or disease. Within a very short period of time, you'll have all the evidence you need.

Chapter 12

THE MILK & APPLE THERAPY
Uniting Two Food Powerhouses

Having personally experienced and witnessed such success with the Milk & Apple Therapy, I wanted to find out why bringing these two foods together has such a powerful effect on our BioChemical Machine.

I was well aware of the beneficial qualities of milk—its high calcium content, many essential vitamins and minerals, as well as the "unidentified factor" that researchers had discovered could retard bone disease and control blood pressure.[37a] *But what was so special about apples?* Although every fruit is extremely healthy, it became obvious that there is something about the chemical makeup of an apple that made it a powerhouse fruit.

I confided my ideas to a colleague who was a great proponent of the BioChemical A&B Method having first hand experienced the way it relieved his arthritis and high blood pressure—and the, almost miraculous, effect it had had on his mother's health.*

He suggested that there might be a correlation between the renowned health of Syrians and the Lebanese and their habit of eating apples. He pointed out that these people were legendary in the Arab world for their strong bones and living to extremely old ages; free of arthritis, heart, liver, and kidney diseases.

I investigated and found that apples are, indeed, a major part of the Lebanese and Syrian diet, which they eat, like most Arabs, with healthy wheat bread, good protein "Neutral" cheeses, vegetables, salads, olives, and other fruits. If they eat cooked meat it is only for special occasions and usually entails the preparation of a whole sheep for a large group of people.

I was intrigued. Everyone knows the old saying, "An apple a day keeps the doctor away." I decided that I wanted to prove it. So I studied and analyzed the chemistry of apples; employing the help of food chemists like Hilka de Groot-Boehlhoff.[38] The result of my research was fascinating. I found that apples are the fruit equivalent of a "jack-of-all trades":

1. Apples are a strong base-building food supplying the body with many important phytochemicals, vitamins, and minerals.

2. Apples stimulate metabolism and their vitamins aid in fat breakdown.

---

*At the beginning of July 1997, his 77-year-old mother was brought into the intensive care unit of a hospital because of dangerously high blood pressure, arteriosclerosis, high blood cholesterol, and calcification of coronary artery vessels. A blood clot in her artery had become life threatening and she was scheduled for surgery on July 16. My colleague insisted on feeding the A&B Method. The result: the surgery, scheduled for July 16, was postponed. On July 29, 1997 the surgery was canceled and she checked out of the hospital.

3. One-fourth of an apple's composition is a substance called *pectin*, which offers the body many healthful benefits:

- Pectin aids digestion.

- Pectin may help reduce cancer and heart disease.

- Pectin is a soluble fiber that lowers artery-clogging LDL blood cholesterol levels by reducing fat absorption.

- Pectin raises levels of HDL: the good cholesterol.

4. Apples regulate the functioning of the intestines and relieve diarrhea.

5. Apples are high in fiber: the roughage that keeps things moving smoothly through your digestive tract.

6. Apples help keep blood sugar levels steady for long periods of time; good news for diabetics, hypoglycemics, and others who are sensitive to blood sugar highs and lows.

7. Apples are loaded with boron: an essential trace element that helps harden bones.

8. A Yale University study showed that apples lowered patients' blood pressure and the level of damaging cholesterol valances and protected the heart and blood vessels.[39]

> **BioChemical Machine Fact:** *One medium apple contains 9 to 10 grams of fiber; a good portion of the 20 to 35 grams you need every day.*

A powerful agent in detoxifying cells…apples also help decompose acid deposits in the tissue—as does whole milk. Whole milk and apples are base-builders. Not only do they help rid the body of poison, but also build up your alkalinity. They're the perfect food marriage: *Apples stimulate the metabolism* so your body can efficiently utilize its vitamins and minerals and elevate your alkaline "savings account."

What's more, a well-balanced blood sugar level that apples help maintain, naturally curbs your appetite. Eating milk and apples in the morning staves off hunger for hours, which is no small consideration when trying to lose weight. Even though our culture is fixated on eating cereals, bread, bagels, and other carbohydrates in the morning—apples and whole milk are a far better breakfast choice. They help build a strong alkaline foundation for the day. Grain carbohydrates, according to our liver's rhythm, should be reserved for the afternoon and evening.

> **BioChemical Machine Fact:** *People with arthritis or osteoarthritis should drink at least one to two glasses of whole milk and eat at least two large apples everyday, such as Golden Delicious, Granny Smith, Empire, Gala, Red Delicious or McIntosh. Other types are equally beneficial.*

As we know from the previous chapter, whole milk's high calcium protects against osteoporosis if you start drinking it early in life.

> **BioChemical Machine Fact:** *Research shows that most people get less than half the calcium they need every day. Professor Claus Leitzmann explains: "The truth is, most people get enough calcium, only their food habits inhibit optimal calcium metabolism." The Osteoporosis Foundation encourages drinking three glasses of milk a day to keep the bones in shape.*[40]

Continuing to get enough calcium is important throughout your life because calcium is regularly drawn from your bones to perform jobs elsewhere in your body and then expelled from the body through urine and perspiration. Calcium must continually be replaced through food.*

Bones are a network of collagen fibers that are impregnated with inorganic salts, especially calcium phosphate. Enveloped within this solid matrix are bone cells, blood vessels, and nerves. The strength of the toughest bone is comparable to reinforced concrete. We need strong bones for overall strength and fitness. Strong, supple bones also aid in the prevention of osteoporosis, a disease in which weakened bones become brittle with age. The disease shows a greater prominence in women, but is also noted in men.

Experiments have confirmed that eating cooked meat—the extremely-bad protein—causes high amounts of calcium to be expelled from the body. Over time, the consumption of bad protein causes over-acidification that can lead to a dismantling of bone substance.

---

*Scientists believe getting calcium from milk is better than calcium supplements.

If the body cannot buffer the acid in the blood, it is forced to mobilize calcium, magnesium, and potassium from its reserves to balance the bases and acids. *And the reserves are in the skeleton.* The skeleton can be de-mineralized over the decades, and the bones will decalcify.

You can avoid acid formation by consuming whole milk and "B" fruits, especially apples, along with calcium-forming foods and base-forming salads, vegetables, and fruits.

You may be surprised to find fruits such as apples, pineapples, apricots, cherries, and oranges in the "B" column, especially since all fruits are not only very healthy, but also vital base-builders (yellow). Placing them in the "B" column is a precaution: these particular fruits contain a short-term (healthy) acid supply and shouldn't be eaten with "A" foods at the same time.

PLEASE NOTE: People with chronic diseases should discuss the Milk & Apple Therapy with their medical doctor. Your doctor will be glad to help you to find out what's right for you.

Healthy people should individually decide how much whole milk they would like to drink. However, you should always eat two (or even more) apples per day. This is one of the best things you can do for your body's savings account; the alkaline reserve.

PART V

KEY FACTORS
IN THE
AGING PROCESS

Chapter 13

MENOPAUSE &
The BioChemical A&B Method

Every woman fears the word menopause. Not because women aren't brave enough to face the reality, but because so many negative things are associated to this change in life. The end of reproductive ability, characterized by irregular menstruation and eventual cessation. Hot flashes, broken or even brittle bones, depression, weakened immune system, pathological fatigue, heavy weight gain, and so many other factors that are considered to be the natural development of your body. But to now be considered old with one's "youthfulness" over may probably be the worst part—besides increasing weight problems. (Don't think that only women have to go through this hardship; men have to go through the same phase. Only most of them don't know this fact. Not only because their "change" is not that *obvious*, but because our culture invented pretty abstract things about men, which are simply not true, but that's another book....)

No wonder why we all believe only hormone replacement therapy might be the answer. And we are terrified! Because we hear so many negative stories about side effects connected to hormone replacement therapy; increased risk of cancer of the uterus and clot formation in the blood vessels leading to possible pulmonary embolism (stroke).

To be honest, it would be sad if our life was considered to be so short—I mean the good life—and everything thought of as "productive" while having lived only half of our lives. The young woman, the grown-up woman, and the wise woman—that's how our ancestors saw life—ancestors who never stepped outside the laws of nature. How could a woman become wise if degenerating bones and other ailments caused severe and daily pain? Wouldn't this distract her from thinking? The truth is that Mother Nature equipped us with many powerful defense and protection mechanisms to live our lives—not to torture ourselves through life.

Even when it comes to hormones, there is a natural replacement in store: By preventing your body from self-poisoning, your suprarenal gland will produce hormones. As thyroid problems can either vanish or at least alleviate with the BioChemical A&B Method, so will menopause symptoms (hot flashes) and consequences (degeneration of bones) and other diseases—and you will have total control over your weight. A side effect of body chemistry balance is that underweight people gain weight and overweight people lose weight.

Because and this must be clear, all these fanatical diets from high-protein to low-carb (which is rather the low-point in human history); from boot camp hype to endless superfluous guru inventions will only work temporarily. *If* you are still young you can torture your body through almost everything, every frenzy that has been around since the 1960s until today. But if you are in your 50s, well, your body's biology will say *"no."* Your guru demons and their "abracadabra" science will begin to haunt you. Pain and chronic disease are the price you'll have to pay for the rest of your life— especially if you are now trying even *harder* to lose weight. *Why?* Because you reached the age when losing weight has become even *more* difficult than ever before (especially when you are another victim of the "Yo-Yo effect).

Yet, at this point in your life, you have a choice. You can repair your body with the BioChemical A&B Method: The suprarenal gland is situated on top of the kidney. It consists of two parts: the cortex and medulla. The cortex (outer part) secretes various steroid hormones, controls salt and water metabolism, and regulates the use of carbohydrates, protein, and fats. The medulla (inner part) secretes the hormones adrenaline and noradrenaline. During stress they cause the heart to beat faster and harder, increase blood flow through heart and muscle cells, dilate airways in the lungs, thus, delivering more oxygen to cells throughout the body, and in general prepare the body to be ready to fight ("flight or fight"). Cortisol is also being produced in the suprarenal gland. Cortisol is the hormone responsible for the glucose [sugar] metabolism. Its main task is to make energy available in the form of "so-called" sugar. For this task, cortisol stimulates the sugar production from the body's own storage (gluconeogenesis), as well as the decomposition from the body's own sugar-depots (glycolysis) and the decomposition of fat for energy (lipolysis). Besides that, the suprarenal gland will

155

produce sexual hormones, be it androgen, estrogen or gestagene. The suprarenal gland marrow is made up primarily of nerve cells. In contrast to other nerve cells, the produced hormones are being released as hormones into the blood. These suprarenal gland marrow products belong to the group of the biogene amines because they are build from amino acids. In addition, the pituitary gland, at the base of the brain (the center for overall coordination of hormone secretion), and the thyroid hormones (that determine the rate of general body chemistry) are able to work as effective as possible due to the BioChemical A&B Method.

In general, our body has a tremendous ability to repair itself, to recover and to replace functions. Of course we will never produce enough hormones to enable our reproductive apparatus pick up its full functions or we could start to reproduce as we did as young women. But at least it provides us with enough hormones to live a happy life with healthy bones, great skin, consistent moods, energy, and joy. In this way we *can* become the "wise woman" (also wise men) who are able to pass on our wisdom to new generations who will profit from our life experiences—instead of listening to the suffering, pain, and sorrow of being "old"—*We will feel like women (and men) in our best years!*

Chapter 14

BREATHING & EXERCISE:
Key Factors in the Aging Process

Physical beauty would be impossible without good health. The skin, our largest organ, is not only one of the vital channels for eliminating toxic wastes, but also the most visible evidence of our beauty. Cosmetic industries have developed hundreds of products to pamper the skin, but there are no miracle creams or beauty products that can keep the human body... "forever young." The body's cells are biologically programmed to age and to die. We cannot prevent our body's aging. However, it is in our power to decelerate the aging process by 20 to 30 years by not poisoning ourselves. It is in *your* power to look and feel, for example, age 50 at age 70.

My mentor, Professor Joachim Seidl, University Munich once said, "Everybody has three ages. The numerical, the biological, and the psychological." Your age does not have to pigeonhole you—you do not have to feel "old" at 50, 60, 70, or even 90. You can look and feel younger than your numerical age because *you* decide what you eat, and what you eat makes a vast difference in the aging process. According to my observations, some individuals are *biologically* 20 to 30 years younger compared to those suffering from a long-standing alkaline deficit. Surely this must influence the state of our psychological age.

"Nature provides a self-governing mechanism for the maintenance of health," said Dr. Hay.[41] In his research he was intrigued by the observations of one Col. Robert McCarrison, of the British Army Medical Service, who was posted in the remote Himalayan region of India during the 1800s.

Dr. McCarrison says that the older men of the tribe looked so much like the younger men that he was often not able to tell the one from the other as they worked in the field or as they swam in the river at the end of the day. They reported living to unbelievable ages; claims which Col. McCarrison, after living among these people for nine years, accepted as genuine.

The older men were apparently as efficient as their much younger counterparts and easily held their own in the strenuous sports of the tribe. [42]

Dr. Hay concluded: "Their life was that of the agrarian spent outdoors at active manual labor. So, oxidation was insured, with little liability of accumulation of the usual unoxidized waste from which we suffer so much in our unwise eating habits."[42]

I made the same observations in Arabia where I met Bedouins who regularly reached their nineties (and beyond). They didn't know arthritis, constipation, allergies, asthma, cancer, arteriosclerosis, diabetes, stroke, or any of our diseases. The oldest living person,

158

actually 135 years of age, was a Bedouin in Lebanon who was videotaped for a story later aired by CNN. His secret, he said, was "sour milk with whole wheat bread every morning." The grandmother of a colleague died in 1994 at 117 years of age. Every morning she ate whole wheat bread and sour milk. Although she didn't know about the BioChemical A&B Method, she *instinctively* lived according to it. Furthermore, she read the newspaper every day and participated actively in society until two years before her death. When she died from the infirmity of her age she was in excellent shape.

I've dedicated most of *The BioChemical Machine* to explain how the foods you eat can empower your body chemistry. But I don't want to entirely neglect two other factors that play a role in keeping you healthy and looking great: exercise and breathing correctly.

Exercise

A huge problem for our generation is that we are deluged with the wrong information: "Don't eat fat, count calories, and work out, work out, work out!" And people believe it. They buy into the notion that heavy-duty exercise will deliver the results they want.

In our efficiency-driven society it has been easy for the $32 billion diet industry to make people believe that the more they work on their bodies the better the results.

So they join fitness clubs or buy expensive equipment and exercise to the point of exhaustion.

Now don't get me wrong...physical exertion is an important part of good health. There's no doubt about it. Chronic inactivity leads to devastating consequences. Exercise—*below* the point of fatigue leads to the important development of your body. However, to exercise *beyond* fatigue leads to deterioration. Everything beyond the fatigue point is damaging because over-exertion produces acid remains that overload the body.

> **BioChemical Machine Fact:** *Excessive exercise creates acid in the body. You can actually feel it happening— the burning pain in your muscles. That's not because you exercised with heroic endurance; it's because acid attacked your nerve endings.*

That's why, later in life, athletes have a greater tendency than most to suffer from conditions like arthritis. You should *always* stop exercising when you feel pain. This is your body signaling to you: enough is enough.

If you haven't exercised for several years then begin slowly with an easy exercise routine and give your body the chance to build up its strength; step by step.

- If you hear music you like—then dance.

- Stretching is great. It strengthens the muscles without undue strain.

- Moderate jogging, a brisk (or ½ hour "normal") walk is fine (with emphasis on "each day"). Both tempos encourage blood circulation and support the work of your BioChemical Machine.

If you are one of the mislead individuals who went through many fad diets and followed a strenuous daily workout…slow down. You'll find that in doing so you will make a huge difference in the quality of your life.

And if you combine moderate exercise with the BioChemical A&B Method, you'll get the results you want.

Breathing

Correct breathing has *much more* impact on our health than generally assumed. Deep breathing exercises massage the abdominal region and by that action improve both blood circulation and the lymphatic system. This, in turn, increases the metabolic rate resulting in enhanced metabolism of fat.

When we sleep we breathe far deeper than when we are awake. It is during sleep that we oxidize our waste matter and eliminate much of it through the lungs. *Why not replicate the same results when we're awake?*

Forced respiration and the perspiration that accompanies exercise expel toxicity from our bodies. The more muscles we use, the more we speed up both respiration and circulation of the blood. Jogging, walking briskly, biking, and swimming are ideal exercises for this reason...as they all call the larger groups of muscles into play.

The benefits of exercise are realized through this massage of the muscles themselves and of the internal organs; through increased respiration, circulation, and perspiration. *In short, you exhale the toxic waste faster.* A combination of moderate exercise and deep breathing is excellent for your BioChemical Machine.

Skin

With the BioChemical A&B Method, the skin also regenerates, which is *not* the case with fad diets. I have seen people who lost weight by dieting but their skin didn't regenerate at the same time. They had nice, new body shapes with the same old skin that tended to sag. This doesn't occur with the A&B way. If you give your body the time to regenerate, as well as observe the rules of your body chemistry—your skin will become more elastic...the sagging effect of stretched skin will be limited. The combination of exercise and the A&B will restore your skin. What is valid for your body muscles is also true for your facial muscles. If, later in life, you choose plastic surgery, it is easier for your doctor to work on healthy skin.

Of course, as you now know, there are many, many wonderful benefits that can be reaped by adapting the BioChemical A&B Method into your day-to-day life. Losing weight and beautiful skin is just a side effect of ridding your body of years of accumulated poison and returning it to its original, balanced state. Not only will you look and feel great, but by balancing your body chemistry you'll also boost your immune system and thwart disease. It can even slow down the effects of the aging process.

Following the BioChemical A&B Method has made a huge difference in the quality of my life—as well as others who have followed it.

Now that you know the truth about the closest companion of your existence—your BioChemical Machine—the decision to make a change is *yours*.

PART VI

PRACTICAL TIPS

Chapter 15

PRACTICAL TIPS:
From Parties to Fast Food Restaurants

The advantage of the BioChemical A&B Method is that you can live and eat normally; regardless of whether you are in the first phase of recovering or have already recouped and are sticking to the A&B. It is easy to follow while shopping in the supermarket or attending parties, weddings, or birthday celebrations. You can easily follow it in restaurants or while traveling. Even fast food restaurants, with their seductive foods, provide enough choices for you to be loyal to the program, to yourself, and to the laws of your body's chemistry. Even if you *do* eat chemically wrong—it's not the end of the world. Simply return to the A&B Method and soon you will be back on track.

In the beginning, before you know the BioChemical A&B chart by heart, I suggest you keep it handy. A quick glance will help you properly negotiate the "pitfalls" at any party and still enable you to enjoy yourself.

Parties, Cookouts, Weddings

Don't listen to silly advice. I recently heard one so-called diet expert recommend eating a yogurt *before* going to a party. This is utter nonsense...another form of unnecessary deprivation. There are always plenty of good food choices at any party. What kind of logic promotes eating before an eating event? I, myself, simply prefer eating correctly *at* the event and enjoy the food and the festivity. However, if you are inclined to eat before going to a party choose anything from the "Neutral" group. These foods will biochemically match anything you might savor at the party.

Since most people drink wine at dinner parties, I suggest choosing foods from the "B" group and, of course, "Neutrals". This means meatballs with tomato sauce; sausages with tomato sauce; roast beef with salad dressing; Swiss cheese; Gouda and other cheeses (mostly below 50% fat); any kind of fruit except for bananas, grapes, figs, and dates; roast venison with cranberry; and salmon with horseradish sauce. With all those delectable, savory choices...why would anyone recommend eating a yogurt before a party—no less someone who is considered a diet expert?

Chicken is often served at parties. If this is your choice, make sure it hasn't been fried with honey-dipped batter. If it has, then simply remove the skin and eat the chicken with mixed salads. You might also find rolled ham, salami, smoked sausages, smoked mackerel, smoked salmon (with horseradish and lemon), herring, and trout. These are fine with salad dressing, pickles, and pickled cucumbers. And, of course, any vegetable or salad with vinegar, oil, and salt is also no problem— see? *No deprivation with the A& B method.*

Potato and pasta salads made with peas, onions, chives, and mayonnaise are party favorites, however if these salads contain pieces of sausages...pass them by. Salads with vinegar, oil, or mayonnaise are fine and even if you choose to eat bread; you can eat it with butter, vegetables, and salads—and of course, salad dressing. If cooked eggs are served, take and crumble only the egg yolk on a slice of bread with a bit of salt...it tastes better than you might expect. Another tasty choice is to mix egg yolk with salad dressing. If you choose bread, potatoes, and noodles; drink beer or sweet wine instead of dry wine and champagne.

If a cookout is on the horizon, you will have to make a choice: either corn with butter and salads *or* meat, such as hamburger, spare ribs, and sausages. If the spare ribs are coated with honey glaze, go ahead, eat them and simply return to the BioChemical A&B Method the following day. After all, sometimes we all need to indulge a little. That next day, simply eat plenty of fruits, salads, and vegetables. *Remember, even if you commit some "chemical mistakes," you can balance them the day after without any lasting problems.*

Restaurants

Eating in restaurants is fairly easy. If you choose a full meal you simply need to omit some food items. If you base your dinner on the "B" column you can start with an hors d'oeuvre such as mozzarella on tomatoes with vinegar, oil, and herbs; artichokes with dressing; eggplant with sour cream; smoked herring, salmon, or mackerel; or smoked ham or bacon (all "Neutrals").

Then, for example, you can continue with a steak topped with sour cream or herb butter; baked tomato; broccoli, green beans and peas (or other vegetables except kale, which is from the "A" column) or for dessert have strawberries with whipped cream. However, omit rice, potatoes, and bread. This is equally valid for chicken, turkey, goose, duck, or lamb chops as the main course. If the duck or chicken is baked with honey—just don't eat the skin.

However, a small problem is presented if your meal includes gravy made with flour. If this is the case, you may see it reflected on the scale the very next day. But again, this is just a small set back. Return to the program the next day and your chemistry will begin to regulate itself once again. After a dinner that is based on "B" column you can eat any kind of "B" fruits, such as apples, oranges, or peaches, but not bananas ("A").

If you choose to eat your dinner based on "A" foods such as spaghetti, rigatoni, or other pasta instead of meat or fish—don't eat it with cooked tomatoes and/or ground meat. But you *can* eat it with cream, peas, mushrooms, or onions. You will see how good it tastes. Moreover, you will realize how good you feel after such a meal. For an hors d'oeuvre with a meal based on "A" foods try some goat or sheep's milk cheese with olives and salads or mozzarella with tomatoes, vinegar, oil, salt, pepper, and herbs. Or you can choose bread with Camembert or salami with mixed salad. You can also enjoy either potato or cauliflower soup.

The same applies if you eat baked potatoes with cottage cheese or sour cream and chives, salads, and vegetables. As a dessert, you can eat banana flambé, cream cheese with raisins, or figs and dates—but not apples, strawberries or other "B" fruits.

Eating in Japanese restaurants is easy. They offer a lot of "Neutral" *raw fish* as in sushi.

Fast Food Restaurants

Eating correctly in fast food restaurants is generally a bit more difficult. The most common foods are usually meat *sandwiches* made with rolls ("A"): roll with hamburger, roll with chicken, roll with roast beef, or roll with fish. Typically, the sandwich or burger will be served with ketchup (cooked tomatoes, strong acid-builder "B") and French fries ("A")—chemically incompatible. However, if you have children, you will **not** be able to avoid fast food restaurants all the time. I admit that fast food really *does* taste seductively good! So, guess what? You can *still* eat according to the BioChemical A&B Method:

- In most restaurants you can order a sandwich with fresh tomatoes, lettuce, onions (or other vegetables), and mayonnaise (and skip the meat and ketchup).

- OR you could eat the French fries or onion rings and bring a meat sandwich home—which you can eat three hours later.

- You can also eat only French fries or onion rings with salads ("A" and "Neutral") and salad dressing, such as oil and vinegar. Just skip the ketchup.

- OR you can eat the other way around: a hamburger (or other cooked meat) with ketchup and all kinds of "Neutral" salads.

If you can find fast food restaurants that offer *pitas*, it will make your life easier because these breads are often stuffed with vegetables and mayonnaise (without chicken or other meat). And this is, of course, perfect. Keep in mind that mayonnaise is "Neutral".

And don't forget, there is nothing wrong with a bagel and cream cheese in the morning; just don't prepare your coffee with milk—use diluted cream instead.

Those who are following the BioChemical A&B Method to maintain their weight can make individual modifications.

The milk shake can be *temporary* trouble. It contains milk and sometimes "B" fruits with sugar from the "A" group. However, even if you *do* succumb to this tasty delight—indulge in the salad bar to balance the meal.

Just in case you can't resist and end up eating an entire hamburger—bun and all—("A", "B", and "Neutral"), simply return to the BioChemical A&B Method as soon as possible.

A hot dog on a bun is probably the most difficult item. Not only because this is clearly matching "A" with "B" "But"—but also, even if you omit the roll and eat *only* the frankfurter with mustard…a hot dog is *not* plain meat. Like other sausages, it contains additives: flour and sugar and as such and may be responsible for quickly putting on pounds. If you *do* indulge in a hot dog from time to time, just get back to the program as soon as possible. ***NOTE: If you are in the process of curing or recovering from a disease, you shouldn't be eating bad or extremely-bad proteins at all.***

One of the most popular fast foods is pizza. There are so many good choices! Pizza with broccoli, mushrooms, onions, peppers, and olives tastes great and they are all chemically perfect. However, *pay careful attention to the cheese*. You should order the "Neutral" cheeses like mozzarella and other cheeses above 60% fat rather than acid-building Parmesan. Also keep in mind that pizza dough is most often made from white flour.

Therefore, avoid pizzas made with tomato sauce ("B"), since the white flour pizza dough is an "A" or order a wheat dough pizza which pizzerias now make or the "all-popular" A&B white pizza.

Falafel is an easy and chemically compatible meal. It is made from flour and beans and can be eaten as offered. It's great with salads. Egyptians always eat beans with onions and radishes (base-builders). That's why they have so few problems digesting beans.

Chinese take-out is also easy because you can eat the meat or fish and vegetables without rice. Or you can eat just the rice with vegetables with no meat. And try ordering brown rice instead of white.

Be aware that most Chinese restaurants use cornstarch to thicken gravies and put sugars in their sweet and sour sauces.

Doughnuts can be eaten on the BioChemical A&B Method, but eating them makes maintaining your weight and avoiding health problems a bit of a challenge. Doughnuts not only include acid-building sugar and white flour but also include ingredients such as milk and eggs. If you eat doughnuts from time to time, remember the three to four-hour waiting period and don't drink your coffee with milk use diluted cream instead.

171

Restaurant pancakes are usually made from flours such as buckwheat, white or whole wheat; all "A" and whole eggs "B"—therefore in conflict. But, if you *cannot* resist, eat them with toppings like honey, bananas, raisins, dates, figs, dried apples, or plums; but NOT with "B" fruits. At home, however, you can make them chemically correct—"Honey Pancakes" are great! (See the A&B Cookbook recipe). But remember the three to four-hour waiting period and don't eat them too often or you will see it on the scale.

Travel

It is just as easy to eat well on an airplane as it is in a restaurant. Airlines typically serve meat with vegetables and "B" or "Neutral" fruits. Simply avoid eating the breads, potatoes, rice, and cookies. Or you can do the reverse: Eat everything, including "A" and/or "Neutral" fruits and not the cooked meats and fish.

It is important to avoid drinking alcohol. Instead, drink a *liter of water* each hour during your flight. Commercial airliners recycle çabin air in an attempt to conserve fuel and the small amount of fresh air brought in is from high altitudes; which is very dry.

If you are traveling in Europe, it's easy to follow the BioChemical A&B Method. In France, Germany, Italy, Spain or Scandinavia you will have no problems. Even in places like Egypt you will find following the A&B Method quite easy. They offer great vegetables with meat and exotic seasonings. You will find fruits as sweet as you have ever tasted. *Just remember, wherever you go in this world you will find chemically matched foods for healthy eating.*

Snacking

The healthiest snacking comes from anything within the "Neutral" column. No waiting periods and, best of all, these foods can be eaten at *any* time. Almost all supermarkets are rich with selections of salads and vegetables. From mushrooms to beets and lettuce to olives. Goat's milk or sheep's milk cheese is fine at any time because they are also "Neutral".

If you want to have something between meals, stick to "Neutrals" since they may be eaten 24 hours a day, 7 days a week without complication. Of course, the best choices are raw vegetables, salads and/or nuts. For example: a couple stalks of raw cauliflower dipped in a *fresh* chunky blue cheese dressing made without preservatives.

In case you want to eat fruits, don't forget the waiting period of three to four hours if your next meal will include food from the "other" group or you intend to eat soon. Keep in mind that some fruits belong to the "B" group and other fruits to the "A" group, but blueberries, avocados and olives are "Neutral".

When eating carrots, don't forget to dip them in oil to make the Vitamin A more readily available to your body.

Walnuts, hazelnuts, almonds, pistachios, cashews, and many other nuts are all "Neutrals" and great for *anytime* snacking. But remember that *peanuts* belong to the "A" group. If you eat nuts (except peanuts) in the afternoon and you would like to add them to a dessert later in the evening...there is no need for any waiting period. They are all "Neutral". But if you eat nuts together with raisins ("A"), you should maintain the three to four hour waiting period in case you are invited for lunch or dinner where you might be served steak, turkey, or other meat or fish.

Other snacks like potato chips, pretzels, or flat breads need to be handled the same way. You eat them like other foods from "A" and keep the waiting period in mind before switching to "B" foods.

Shopping

You don't need to buy your foods for the BioChemical A&B Method in specialty or "health-food" stores. You just need to choose the right foods according to your body's chemistry. The goal for healthy eating is easily achieved with foods readily available at your favorite supermarket. However:

(1) Don't buy low-fat or fat-free products, because they typically contain sugar, corn syrup and plenty of additives to make them "tasty." The sugar will disturb your body's chemistry—and many important vitamins and minerals are absent in these items.

(2) Avoid buying prepared foods. They are full of chemicals, flour and sugars that will upset your body chemistry.

(3) If you buy canned foods...check the labels. If there is too much sugar in a product...avoid it. If you can make your own mayonnaise at home... then do it! (See the A&B Cookbook)

(4) Buy whole wheat, rye, or other whole grain bread *instead* of white bread. Remember that vitamins from the grains are removed from white bread.

The price difference is extremely small and you will automatically eat less because your system is satisfied. Place the bread in your refrigerator to keep it fresh. Buy extra and freeze it!

(5) Wash vegetables and fruits with warm water to remove as many pesticides (poisons) as possible. Don't forget that these dangerous chemicals are intended to kill animals and insects and some are extremely resistant to washing.

(6) Organic foods (biological/ecological agriculture) such as vegetables and fruits are good because you theoretically avoid pesticides and other poisons. Supermarkets are increasingly offering organic foods. But be careful when shopping for organic foods as they are not yet regulated and some companies get away with selling non-organic foods at "organic" prices; *look for certified organic labeling.*

Cooking

When cooking you should keep a copy of the BioChemical A&B Chart close at hand. After deciding what to prepare, verify that all the ingredients fit together chemically.

The A&B Method is NOT about deprivation or quantity but about basic BioChemical principles.

- Beware when recipes call for white flour. Use "Neutral" whole wheat flour or soy flour when preparing foods from the "B" column.
- Don't cook your chicken in commercial barbecue sauce or prepared breadcrumb mixes.

175

- For cakes and cookies, use cream diluted with water instead of milk and only use the egg yolk rather than the whole egg (See BioChemical A&B Method recipes). Yeast is "Neutral" and therefore perfect for baking cookies and cakes.
- Eat raw vegetables as frequently as possible. If you need to cook vegetables…steam them to retain as many vitamins as possible. Whenever you eat acid-building foods such as cooked meat, cooked fish, sausages and cheeses below 50% fat; try to eat them with fresh fruits (but not bananas, grapes, figs and dates on the "A" column). It tastes good and balances the acid-alkaline levels in our bodies.

A Tip for Working People

If you bring your lunch to work, be sure to include either fruits from the "B" group or any kind of vegetable salad. You can eat the A&B Method Power Salad (see recipe in cookbook) and "B" fruits with cottage cheese, goat or sheep's milk cheese, feta, mozzarella; or cream cheese, Roquefort, ricotta, and anything from the "Neutral" group. Many of these foods are readily available at salad bars in the local supermarket or deli.

Be careful with ready-mixed salad dressings… especially during the first phase of detoxifying your system. Most of them contain sugar, flour, corn syrup and chemicals. However, there *are* plenty of fresh dressings and dips available—*just check the labels*. If you want to play it safe…use vinegar or lemon with olive oil, sea salt and pepper.

Chapter 16

QUESTIONS AND ANSWERS
From A to Z

- ALCOHOL *"What about alcohol? Do I have to stop drinking, or can I have an occasional glass of wine or beer?"*
  - o BEER is slightly acid-building and on the boundary of being "Neutral"—i.e., moderate base-building. You can drink it with any food from the "Neutral" and "A" groups.
  - o DRY WINE is *moderately* acid-building and you can drink it with any food from the "Neutral" and "B" groups.
  - o CHAMPAGNE and SWEET WINE are also *strong* acid-builders, but you can drink them with any food from the "Neutral" or "B" groups.
  - o RYE WHISKEY and GIN belong to the "Neutral" group, despite being strong acid-builders. *(Acid-building alcohol should be avoided if your health doesn't allow it. If you have health problems, you should discuss the amounts with your doctor.)*

- BEANS *"What about beans?"*

Beans are believed to be difficult to digest. But if this were *really* true, how could this food item be the national dish of so many countries? Until the turn of the last century, beans were the national dish not only in Arabia, but also in Europe, Africa, Asia, and Middle and South America until our "economic miracle" forever changed our eating habits. Being "National Dish" automatically means that the food must be healthy, must taste good, and must be inexpensive. The truth is that all *fresh beans*, as well as peas or lentils are all part of the food group "legume" and are base-builders *before drying*. Acid-forming dried beans become alkaline-forming when sprouted. Alkaline-forming dried soybeans, however, increase their alkaline dramatically when sprouted. Among 500 different types of beans, there are the well-known brown, white, and Garbanzo beans (chickpeas) and also the less-known fava beans. The small and skinless fava beans are the Egyptian national dish (see A&B Cookbook recipe "Ramses Beans") that also includes Garbanzo beans and lentils. This dish is the backbone of the Egyptian farmers' nutrition and they are probably one of the healthiest people on earth. The Egyptians don't have any problem digesting the beans because they *prepare* them properly. The Egyptians *soak* the beans in water for at least 3-4 hours; this prepares them (unknowingly) for a chemical process that makes digestion easier. *Moreover, the Egyptians are eating the Ramses Beans the way they ought to be eaten:* with base-builders, wheat bread and olive oil. They always eat their dish either with several raw onions (prepared with vinegar, pepper, salt, and cumin, crushing the onions gently with their hand for the sake of the spices) or with only fresh radishes or special salads; such as the Ramses Salad. The Egyptians, like all Arabs, rarely eat kidney beans, white and brown beans or beans in cans. These beans require an even more complicated preparation process and are, ultimately, difficult to digest. But the main reason for the preference of Arabian connoisseurs is most certainly that fava beans have a particular taste that makes Ramses Beans so delicious.

• CALORIE COUNTING *"Should I count calories?"*
No! The idea of "calories" stems from the time when the steam engine was born: put in coal and out comes energy. At that time people believed that it must be the same with food. The idea is simplistic and limited in scope: we are *not* steamboats that are powered with steam engines needing to be fueled—we *are* a BioChemical Machine, but one that works upon the laws of our body's own chemistry with compatible foods as our fuel.

• CANNED FOOD *"What about canned food?"*
Canned fruits and vegetables are *not* recommended because most of the vitamins are destroyed during the cooking process. Many canned fish products contain water and salt; if you are healthy this is okay from time to time. The same is true for canned meat and sausages. Avoid canned food that contains sugar, corn, and flour.

• CEREAL AND MILK *"Can I add milk to my cereal?"*
If you usually add milk to your cereal (hopefully without sugar)—instead of using milk, try yogurt or

cream; plain or diluted with water. It's the same taste—with a different chemistry. This is also recommended for baking cakes, cookies, and sweets; replace the milk with cream diluted with spring water.

- CHEESE *"What about cheese? Is it true that I should avoid dairy products?"*

Definitely not! Cheese with a fat content above 60% is a healthy "Neutral". It can be eaten with bread (preferably wheat bread) and anything from the "A", "B", and, of course the "Neutral" groups. But cheese with a fat content below 50% ("B") is an acid-builder. Limit the amounts of cheese below 50% fat, along with American processed cheese and pasteurized or processed cheese foods. These "B" cheeses can be eaten with anything from the "B" and "Neutral" groups, but not with bread, pizza, noodles, or anything from "A". Try to eat cheese below 50% fat with "B" fruits or "Neutral" fruits. Eliminate low-fat/fat-free cheese products; not only are they lacking the good taste of regular cheeses, but they also contain unhealthy and/or incompatible acid-building sugar and artificial additives. If you are in the process of losing weight or if your cholesterol is high, restrict not only cheese below 50% fat, but also cheese above 60% fat.

- CHEWING *"Why is chewing so important?"*

Chewing your carbohydrates, such as bread, potatoes, noodles extremely well activates the enzyme amylase for digestion. "A" column carbohydrates should be chewed 25 to 40 times according to the latest research. Saliva is necessary in the first step of carbohydrate digestion (and its action) due to the enzyme amylase.

- CHOCOLATE *"Is it true that chocolate makes you fat?"*

No! Yet, "A" white sugars and brown sugars products are *not really* recommended. However, even unhealthy carbohydrates *(gray)* are not as damaging as the extremely-bad proteins. Therefore, "A" chocolate and sweets may be eaten moderately with other foods from the "Neutral" and "A" columns, but *not* with items from the "B" column. You will find a number of recipes for chemically correct, great-tasting cakes, cookies, and other sweets in the cookbook section.

- COFFEE

See Milk and Coffee

- DIPS and SALAD DRESSING

Although ready-made food is *not* recommended due to chemical additives and fillers like sugar, flour, and corn syrup—there are plenty of salad dressings and dips available which are fresh and produced *without* preservatives. Just read the labels first and you'll find creamy Italian garlic dips, Blue Cheese dips, and others in your supermarket. However, as long as dips and salad dressings *with preservatives* are used on your A&B salad or vegetables such as cauliflower, broccoli, spinach, onion, and carrots…minor chemicals that might be added won't make a major difference. The most important point is to get as many fresh vegetables and salads into your system as possible.

- DRIED FRUITS *"What about dried fruits?"*

Dried unsulfured fruits are great. Dried *sulfured* fruits such as apples and pears are less recommended; but acceptable.

- EGGS *"What about eggs?"*

Do not eat whole eggs more than three times a week; avoid egg whites (albumin/sulfur-containing bad protein)—but *egg yolks* are healthy. The egg yolk is a good "Neutral" protein and the whole egg belongs to the "B" group. Spread wheat bread with mayonnaise and crumble the cooked egg yolk over your bread, or mash the egg yolk and add mayonnaise to a spreading consistency. You will be surprised how delicious it tastes.

- FATS *"What about healthy fats?"*

Butter and natural oils such as olive oils, sunflower oils, flaxseed oils, soy oils, and sesame oils are healthy. A total of 60 to 80 grams of fat for moderately active men and women and teenage girls and boys is a healthy daily allowance. However, the amount of healthy fats should be individually adjusted to the activity of a person. People with health problems should discuss the amount with their medical doctor. Avoid industrialized oils.

- FAT-FREE/LOW-FAT PRODUCTS *"Will eating fat-free or low-fat products help me to lose weight?"*

Definitely not! If this were the case, it would be easy to lose weight because you would just need to avoid eating fat. Let's face it: how much (healthy) fat can you eat over the course of a day in order to reach a total of 60 to 80 grams, which is the recommended amount for a healthy and moderately active person? So why would you need low-fat/fat-free products which deprive your cells from vital vitamins, and moreover, contain sugar and artificial additives, which interfere with your body's chemistry and metabolism. These additives are not only unhealthy, but above all, interfere with the A&B principles. Therefore, completely eliminate low-fat and fat-free products from your menu. Replace them with healthy oils and their vital minerals and vitamins, such as vitamin E. *Instead* of eating low-fat or fat-free products...*eat,* for example, cauliflower. It is high in pantothenic acid and *it demolishes fat.* Cauliflower plays a central role in the biochemical reactions within the body.

- FISH (COOKED) *"What about cooked fish?"*

Cooked fish is an acid-builder. Try to eat the fish with "B" or "Neutral" fruits, vegetables, and salads. But check with the A&B Chart. You will find that there are smoked herring, smoked mackerel, smoked trout, smoked salmon, and marinated white herring in the "Neutral" group, which taste great and are chemically compatible with the A&B Method. However, even cooked fish is better for us than cooked meat.

- HONEY *"Is honey healthy?"*

Yes! Pure natural honey (cold rinsed) is highly recommended. Other honey is less recommended but acceptable. Honey ("A") may be eaten with any other food from the "A" and "Neutral" groups, but not with foods from the "B" group.

- MARGARINE *"Is margarine better than butter?"*
Although it is a "Neutral" vegetable product, the use of commercial margarine is *not* recommended. The heating process, used in making margarine, breaks hydrogen bonds and creates a product that causes rancidity and hardening in the tissues. Butter (a moderate base-builder) is much more digestible than margarine and is therefore more highly recommended.

- MAYONNAISE *"Is it true that mayonnaise makes me fat?"*
Not at all! Mayonnaise belongs to the "Neutral" group and may be eaten like all fats and oils with "A", "B", and/or "Neutral" foods.

- MEAT (COOKED) *"What about cooked meat?"*
Meat is a strong acid-builder. You should eat it only from time to time. However, if you eat cooked/fried meat, then try to eat it with vegetables, salads, and fruits. However, there are "Neutral" meat products such as bacon, smoked ham, rolled ham, cured meat, and dried meat, which not only taste great, but their chemistry suits the body's chemistry.

- MILK *"Will I get diarrhea from drinking milk!"*
You might go through the so-called Healing Crisis, while the body works hard to get rid of the body toxins. You might experience diarrhea, headache, and shooting pains. The reaction differs according to age or the progress of a disease. After approximately one week on the A&B Method, the body begins to better tolerate the milk.

- MILK and COFFEE *"What about milk in my coffee?"*

If you eat wheat bread with honey and some cottage cheese and at the same time you drink coffee, use cream or cream diluted with spring water instead of milk in the coffee. But if you eat food from the "B" or "Neutral" groups you can drink your coffee with regular milk. However, black coffee is "Neutral" and in the summer is great as a cold beverage.

- READY-MADE FOOD *"What about ready-made food?"*

Limit (*preferably eliminate*) ready-made foods because of artificial additives, sugar, corn syrup, corn starch, fructose, bread crumbs, bleached flours, acetic acid, cooked tomatoes, and many chemicals added to these foods.

- SALAD DRESSINGS See Dips.

- SWEETENING *"How should I sweeten foods, coffee and tea?"*

Sweeten with sugar substitutes, fresh fruits, or pure honey (cold rinsed). Other honey is less recommended but acceptable. Since honey is in the "A" group it may be eaten with other foods from the "A" and "Neutral" groups, but should not be added to foods from the "B" group.

- SOY PRODUCTS *"What about soy products?"*

Prior to processing, soybeans are strong base-builders. However, soy flour (made of soy beans), soy imitations, and soy ready-mixtures turn into moderate acid-builders (*white* on the A&B Chart) after processing.

- SOY SPROUTS/SOY SAUCE

Soy sprouts and soy oil are in the "Neutral" group and base-builders (*yellow* on the A&B Chart). They are indeed healthy. This is also true for soy sauce.

- TOFU *"Is it true that tofu has the power to cure cancer?"*

Tofu (made from soy beans) is a high-grade protein food item, however in the "Neutral" group like all leguminous plant foods—beans, lentils, and peas which are *white* on the A&B Chart. (Please read Chapter 9.)

- WEIGHT *"Do I need to weigh myself every day?"*

You don't need to weigh yourself every day. Just let it go. There are phases during the healing crisis when you won't see any change on the scale. Since your body is getting rid of its poison your weight will regulate itself. If you are overweight; you will lose weight. If you are underweight; you will gain weight. At the beginning, I suggest sticking with the A&B principles not interrupting the important work of the body's chemistry until you have reached your goal. It is best to weigh yourself only once a week.

- WRONG EATING *"What if I strayed from the A&B Method?"*

If you already detoxified your body and your acid-alkaline balance is in good shape (and you are losing weight) the time may come when you can't resist "eating wrong." For example: you eat a complete meal in a fast food restaurant, such as hamburger on a roll and French fries with a milkshake (which is from the

"A" group and "B" group at the same time). Don't worry. You just need to go back to the BioChemical A&B Method and you will soon be back on track towards health and perfect weight. A detoxified body can easily deal with occasional mistakes every now and then. In the event you start to feel badly, immediately eat some raw vegetables, salads, and/or fruits to increase your alkaline levels. The best vegetables to use for this purpose (besides "Neutral" and "B" fruits) are raw vegetables and salads, such as root vegetables, carrots, (adding a few drops of oil to make it easier for your body to utilize the valuable Vitamin A) turnips, beets, and all sorts of top vegetables, such as spinach, sprouts, beet tops, chard, celery, onion tops, watercress, broccoli, cauliflower, or any green vegetable that contains juice. These vitamins and minerals will enable your metabolism to do its job. You will soon feel better.

PART VII

GETTING STARTED:
TURNING THE A&B METHOD
INTO PRACTICAL USE

Chapter 17

GETTING STARTED
A One-Day Suggested Example

While sharing the wonders of the BioChemical A&B Method with family, friends, and other interested parties over the past seven years I was often asked, "What is the best way to get started?" I realized that, similar to other life challenges, getting started was the toughest part. Therefore, I've included this one-day example to help you along. I am confident that once you begin…the rest of the program will quickly fall into place. Upcoming chapters will provide you with similar quick-start, four-week examples for both LEVEL ONE and LEVEL TWO.

BREAKFAST

You can eat either:

A. Milk and apples and other "B" fruits. Although you might not think this is a complete and healthy breakfast—*it is.* It will satisfy your nutritional requirements and prevent you from becoming hungry over the next three to four hours. Try apples in bite-size pieces with yogurt on top.
B. Cereal with raisins, bananas, and cream (diluted with water), or plain yogurt (can be sweetened with a sugar substitute) and buttermilk.
C. Wheat bread topped with one of the following: cottage cheese; cream cheese and honey; bacon and goat's cheese; butter, fresh tomatoes, and sea salt.
D. Bagel with cream cheese.
E. Scrambled (whole eggs) with bacon (without bread). –OR-
   Scrambled *egg yolks* with smoked bacon *(not fried!)* with bread.

There are no limits when you use your imagination to create the perfect BioChemical breakfast.

- Remember the BioChemical A&B principle: Don't eat "A" foods with "B" foods.

- If you need to drink coffee then use "Neutral" cream instead of "B" milk, especially if your breakfast includes "A" cereal or "A" wheat bread.

Remember, coffee is a strong acid-builder. Furthermore, coffee directly affects your heart and circulatory system and interferes with your hormones. Tea also affects the brain and central nervous system, although much more slowly than coffee. Black tea with its minerals, fluorine, potash, and manganese is a better choice and herbal tea is the *best* choice.

FROM BREAKFAST TO LUNCH

In the beginning, you may sometimes find yourself hungry in between meals. Don't fret; this is because your body's chemistry is still undergoing changes. The good news is you *can* eat in between meals as long as you choose foods from the "Neutral" column like mozzarella cheese on tomatoes, a mushroom salad, or any fresh vegetables or lettuce. These can be eaten anytime, 24 hours a day; seven days a week. Salads and vegetables are great. Don't laugh, but even a cooked egg yolk (without the egg white!) with a little bit of mayonnaise is a tasty snack that can be eaten on the A&B Method.

LUNCH

Lunch will depend on your particular circumstances. However, some great choices include:

A. All leafy salads including the A&B Power Salad (see Chapter 18 and cookbook).
B. Mozzarella with tomatoes, basil, vinegar, olive oil, sea salt, and pepper.
C. Meat, fried chicken, sausages, or fish with vegetables, salads and "B" fruits.

Cooked tomatoes or cooked spinach matches perfectly with these meals. Gravies made with cream are also great. Parmesan cheese is fine. Lunch may also be accompanied by unsweetened wine. In order to compensate for the bad protein consumption, you should try to eat a base-building apple, melon or any "B" fruit like peaches, grapefruit, kiwi, or oranges. NO "A" fruits such as bananas, figs or dates. Save them for the evening.

FROM AFTERNOON TO DINNER

Vegetables, salads, or any other "Neutral" foods can be eaten at any time. However, if you plan to eat pizza, potatoes, rice, noodles or anything else from the "B" column for dinner...remember the three to four hour waiting period. And, if you know that you are going to eat carbohydrates at dinner time, then you can also eat raisins or bananas or play it safe by choosing "Neutrals".

DINNER

Since The A&B Method is *not* a diet you can create meals from whatever you like…as long as the foods are chemically compatible. Your culinary fantasies have no boundaries. Here are just a few examples:

A. A&B Pizza with A&B Sauce. (See "A" lunches and Dinners.)
B. Baked potatoes with olive oil, herbs and cream cheese, and/or butter with herbs and vegetables and/or salad.
C. Fried (natural) rice or (whole wheat) noodles.
D. A&B Power Salad (see next chapter) with whole wheat bread, potatoes, rice, noodles and/or any "Neutral" cheese.
E. Ramses Beans and Ramses Salad or Lentils or Lentil soup. (See next chapter.)
F. "Neutral" smoked ham with wheat bread and salad.
G. A&B-Burger® or A&B Sandwiches (see A&B Cookbook) with mayonnaise, tomatoes, lettuce, onions, or Camembert, salami, feta and much more.

Beer belongs to the "A" group and goes well with all the above.

If you find you're still hungry before bedtime… have an evening snack of nuts, raisins, honey, carrots with olive oil, cauliflower with dips (see A&B Cookbook in Part VIII), or anything else from the "Neutral" column. Just keep in mind:

- Whenever you want to switch between "A" and "B" foods, it is best to wait three to four hours.

- Even if you are healthy, remember the BIG SEVEN ESSENTIALS—and the fact that your liver doesn't like working overtime at night.

Chapter 18

FOUR-WEEK EXAMPLE MENU
For Healthy People

LEVEL ONE

Early in 2001, I was approached by the editors of the popular German publication *Petra Magazine*. They indicated that they were familiar with my research and asked if I might be interested in putting the A&B Method to a public test! Being completely confident in the program's simple effectiveness, I immediately jumped at the opportunity. To get them started as quickly as possible, I created a four-week example menu for LEVEL ONE. I have included that exact example in this chapter.

In the June 2001 issue, the editors reported on the BioChemical A&B experience.

Healthy weight loss! Petra shows you the main points of the new A&B Method....The new A&B Method in Eleonora De Lennart's book is a work of genius, as well as scientifically sound. During her research, De Lennart worked together with physicians, professors, and scientists..."It is," says De Lennart, "about the perfect match of food chemistry and body chemistry." If one disregards the chemistry, the body is going to be over-acidified, and, as a result, poisoned. The consequences are overweight and loss of energy...Instead, if one provides the body with base-surplus nourishment, not only will the alkaline reserve—a buffer system—build up, but healthy chemistry will also be restored.

This all sounds scientific and complicated. But in practice this is not the case at all. We [at Petra*] have tried the A&B with success (15.5 lbs. in three weeks) with a little bit of training and a lot of fun. And the great part: one may eat potatoes, spaghetti, pizza and desserts, yet nevertheless one loses weight.*

Don't worry if you can't follow the rules exactly because you have been invited out or you're going to McDonald's. Simply have one or two "clean" meals. Even alcohol is allowed...Frozen fruits and vegetables are fine.

If you want to know more about this method or want to know more about the delicious A&B menus, read The BioChemical Machine.

Petra Magazine, www.petra.de., June 2001

In addition, Mrs. Bigs Moeller, director of the Health and Beauty Department of *Petra*, wrote me a letter on September 2, 2002, confirming, upon my request, her thoughts about the four-week example. She responded:

Dear Eleonora: We recommended in our article [June 1, 2001, No. 6-01] the A&B as a basis for a whole nutrition-philosophy and/or as a normal four-week program. Kindest regards, Bigs Moeller.

The program designed for and tested by the editors of *Petra* was drawn from the basic principles of the LEVEL ONE chart. Simply put, healthy individuals following the LEVEL ONE chart will successfully rid their BioChemical Machine of the poisons that trigger acid formation. Like the *Petra* editors, you will soon increase your *alkaline reserve*, experience improved health and vitality, and as a bonus side effect, you will correct your weight.

BioChemical Machine Fact: The A&B Method requires that people who have already developed chronic diseases need to follow the ratio of 80% base-builders and not more than 20% healthy acid-builders as prescribed in LEVEL TWO. This will be outlined in more detail in Chapter 19.

So, if your health status follows the requirements for the LEVEL ONE chart and you want to start sampling all the delicious meals you can enjoy while following the A&B Method continue Chapter 18.

DAY ONE

BREAKFAST:

Milk & Apples

1–2 glasses of whole milk or yogurt with a minimum of 2 large apples (or 3 medium apples), or any kind of "B" fruits from the "Neutral" or "B" column (bananas, figs, and dates are "A"). Apples are high in fiber. A medium apple contains 9 to 10 grams of fiber, a good portion of the 20 to 35 grams you need every day. One glass of milk (250 ml) contains 8 grams fat, a fragment of the 60 to 80 grams fat that are healthy for a moderately active person. By drinking whole milk (moderate base-builder) and eating apples (strong base-builders) you are building a strong alkaline foundation for *the day.*

ALTERNATIVE:

Bagel with cream cheese
    OR
Wheat bread topped with cottage cheese
Cream cheese and honey
Bacon and goat's cheese
Butter, fresh tomatoes and sea salt
    OR
Scrambled (whole eggs)
    with either:
Smoked bacon (without bread), OR scrambled egg yolks with smoked bacon (not fried!), with bread;
    OR

Classic Cereal Breakfast: Large bowl of cereal (whole grain, without sugar), with either yogurt or sour cream
  OR
Cream (diluted with spring water). May be served with bananas, blueberries, and/or raisins or dates, dried figs, honey, and/or all kinds of "Neutral" nuts, including peanuts from the "A" column.
  OR
Whole grain toast with butter and honey, or with butter or mayonnaise and/or any "Neutral" cheese above 60% fat, (such as cream cheese, cottage cheese, Camembert, goat's milk cheese), topped with chives, tomatoes, onions or any other vegetable and herb; or any "Neutral" meat/sausage, such as smoked or rolled ham.

- Drink tea, herbal tea, water or coffee. Instead of milk, *put cream diluted with spring water* in your coffee if you eat bread, cereal, or a bagel.
- You can drink your coffee with regular milk if you eat eggs. However, the base-building cream *neutralizes the acid-building* coffee.

WHAT ABOUT SNACKS?

If you want to have something between meals, you may eat "Neutrals", 24 hours a day; 7 days a week. Try mozzarella cheese on tomatoes, mushroom salad, or any fresh vegetables, lettuce, or salads. Also, a couple stalks of raw cauliflower dipped in chunky blue cheese dressing, fresh and made without preservatives—not only tastes good but also works wonders.

And, of course, fruits! "Neutral" or "B" cheese with "B" or "Neutral" fruits taste delicious. Keep in mind that some fruits belong to "B," others to "A," but blueberries are "Neutral".

LUNCH:

There is no limit to the number of vegetables, salads, sprouts, and herbs you can have at lunch. You don't need to add ALL of the following suggested vegetables to your A&B Power Salad, but it's more powerful if you do. By eating so many different vegetables and salads, you add tremendous power to your metabolism.

A&B POWER SALAD*

Lettuce (romaine, iceberg, limestone, red leaf, watercress, or any other lettuce, broken into bite-size pieces)
Tomatoes, sliced or diced into cubes
Cucumber, sliced or diced into cubes
Carrots, chopped or sliced
Cauliflower, chopped
Broccoli, chopped
White and/or red cabbage, chopped
Sprouts/soy sprouts
Spinach, chopped
Onions, sliced or diced into cubes
Scallions, sliced
Parsley, chopped
Chive, chopped
Oil to taste (olive, flaxseed, sesame, etc.)
Apple vinegar (opt: balsamic) or fresh lemon juice to taste
Salt (sea salt, herb salt, Bio-salt) to taste
Pepper to taste

1. Cut up vegetables. In a large bowl, combine all vegetables.
2. In a small bowl, combine oil, vinegar, salt, pepper, and chives (or OPTIONAL salad dressings, such as chunky blue cheese dressing or mayonnaise dip. See A&B Cookbook in Part VIII).
3. Pour dressing over salad.

IF YOU WORK and bring your food from home, then eat either cheeses/mozzarella with apples; any fruit from the "Neutral" or "B" group; chicken with oranges; Chef Salad; or any kind of salad; such as the A&B Power Salad.

You can eat your salads and fruits with cottage cheese, goat or sheep's milk cheese, feta, mozzarella, cream cheese, Roquefort, ricotta, Camembert, or anything from the "Neutral" group. You will realize that you can buy almost the same foods at salad bars in supermarkets, delis, and restaurants.

- The A&B Power Salad can be eaten with "Neutral" cheese (cottage, ricotta, Camembert, cream Brie, etc.) or "B" cheese (Cheddar, Colby, Gouda, etc.), "Neutral" meat (salami, smoked or cured ham, dried meat, etc.) or "B" meat (cooked meat, cooked sausages, etc.), "Neutral" fish (smoked, marinated, or raw fish), or "B" fish (cooked fish). If you eat the A&B Power Salad with "B" or "Neutral" meat, "B" or "Neutral" fish, or "B" or "Neutral" cheese, you should eat it with "B" fruits and, of course, with anything from the "Neutral" column.

- The A&B Power Salad can also be eaten with "A" foods, such as (steamed or baked) potatoes, rice, pasta, and, of course, all kinds of whole grain breads, such as whole wheat, rye, potato, oat, etc. (see Cookbook, A&B Sandwiches). But remember Essential #5, the biological liver rhythm in Chapter 5. Your liver doesn't like "A" food before late afternoon/ early evening. If you choose to eat the A&B Power Salad with wheat bread, potatoes, rice, or pasta, you may also eat bananas, grapes, figs, dates, nuts, raisins, honey, and anything from the "Neutral" group. In this case you can choose any "A" or "Neutral" DESSERT from the cookbook.

HELPFUL TIP: *Most people quickly tire of cutting up vegetables day in and day out. In order to have this vital food available any time you are hungry you should prepare a huge bowl of raw vegetables sufficient for a couple of days. Non-leafy vegetables don't perish quickly and can be kept refrigerated in a sealed container for several days. Chop or slice carrots and white and/or red cabbage and prepare cauliflower and broccoli according to your taste. Put chopped onions in a separate sealed bowl, so that your refrigerator will not smell. Prepare (wash and cut) only a limited amount of fresh leafy greens/lettuce, since they perish very quickly. When you come home, you just need to take a bit from every bowl and mix with oil, vinegar, and sea salt.*

Snacks from Lunch to Dinner:
If you ate your lunch with "Neutrals" you have no restrictions. If you ate your lunch with cooked meat, cooked sausages, or cooked fish ("B" group foods), you can snack on "B" or "Neutral" fruits. But don't forget the waiting period of three to four hours in regard to the pizza ("A" group) you might eat for dinner. If you ate your lunch with potatoes, bread, rice, or pasta, you may snack on fruits from the "A" and "Neutral" groups or anything from the "Neutral" group with emphasis on base-builders.

DINNER:

A&B Four Seasons White Pizza

2 cups whole wheat flour
1 tablespoon yeast
1 1/2 cups water
1 tablespoon salt
1 cup Ricotta cheese
1/2 cup heavy cream
3 cloves garlic
1 teaspoon dried parsley
1 teaspoon basil
1 teaspoon oregano
2 cups mozzarella, shredded
2 tablespoons olive oil
1 tablespoon butter
1 tablespoon olive oil
Broccoli, small pieces (quantity to taste)
Cauliflower, quantity to taste
Mushrooms, sliced, quantity to taste
1/2 eggplant, sliced 3/4 inch
1 large onion, sliced into rings
Olives, quantity to taste

A&B Pizza Sauce: In a food processor, combine Ricotta cheese, garlic, cream, oregano, parsley, dried basil. Process until a paste forms. Slowly add oil; set aside.

A&B Pizza Dough: In a medium mixing bowl combine flour, yeast, oil, salt, and water. Stir mixture; knead with your hands until dough is firm but moist (if necessary, add more water, 1 tablespoon at a time). Let dough rest for 1 hour.

1. Knead dough again with your hands. Cover and let rise for 20 minutes in a warm place.
2. Preheat oven to 350°F. Sprinkle whole wheat flour over greased baking sheet. Roll out dough and place on baking sheet.
3. Spread pizza sauce evenly over dough. Top with broccoli, cauliflower, mushrooms, eggplant, onions, and olives. Sprinkle mozzarella evenly over pizza. Place baking sheet on lowest shelf in oven (or the floor of a gas oven) and bake until crust is firm and golden brown, 15 to 20 minutes. Serve warm.

205

OTHER DINNER OPTIONS:

Ramses Salad
With Whole Wheat Bread or Whole Wheat Pita Bread

5–6 fresh hot peppers, such as jalapeno
2–3 large tomatoes
1 head of lettuce
6 large cloves of garlic
2 large onions
1 tablespoon coriander
1 bunch cilantro
1 tablespoon cumin
Salt and pepper to taste
1/2 cup vinegar and
1/2 cup olive oil

In a food processor, combine pepper, tomatoes, onions, lettuce, garlic, salt, pepper, vinegar, oil, and herbs. Process until well blended to form a pulp. *TIP: Put the remaining Ramses Salad in a jar. Cover with olive oil, 2-inches above pulp. Refrigerate for later use.*

A&B-BURGER® or A&B SANDWICH

(See A&B Cookbook). Or try whole wheat bread with butter, mayonnaise, bacon, and/or cheese above 60% fat (cream cheese, Camembert, Brie, cottage cheese, or any other "Neutral" cheese) with raw vegetables and dill spears

DESSERT:

You can choose any "A" or "Neutral" dessert from the cookbook, such as:

Banana Cream

2 pounds bananas
2 cups heavy cream, whipped
1/2 teaspoon vanilla
1/4 cup almonds, minced
Raisins
Honey to taste
In a processor, combine bananas, honey with whipped cream, 1/2 teaspoon vanilla, and honey. Process until mixture is firm. Garnish with raisins; refrigerate.

Snacks From Dinner To Bedtime:
Choose anything from the "Neutral" group with an emphasis on base-building nuts, honey, vegetables, salads and "A" fruits.

DAY TWO

BREAKFAST: Same as Day One
LUNCH:

Broccoli Milanese*   2 servings

4 stalks broccoli, washed and stems cut off
2 tablespoons butter
2 teaspoons fresh lemon juice
Seasoning to taste

1. Cut each broccoli stem into individual florets. Place in vegetable steamer over boiling water until tender, covered, for 7 minutes.
2. In a small saucepan, melt butter. Combine with lemon juice. Pour sauce over hot broccoli. Season to taste.

COMPATIBLE with "A", "B", and "Neutral" foods
*Optional for Working People: Same as Day One

DINNER:

New Potatoes Marseilles   2 servings

5 small red-skinned potatoes, unpeeled
(Alternative: 1–2 New Jersey potatoes, russet potatoes or other type)
2–3 tablespoons butter, melted
1/4 cup fresh parsley, chopped
Salt and pepper to taste

1. In a vegetable steamer, bring water to a boil. Place washed, potatoes over boiling water. Cook until tender. Remove from heat. Place potatoes in a large bowl. Let stand until potatoes are cool enough to handle.
2. Cut unpeeled potatoes into quarter-inch slices. Place on baking sheet and sprinkle evenly with butter. Sprinkle with seasoning and place as close as possible to heat of broiler until crusty and golden.

COMPATIBLE with "A" and "Neutral" foods
OTHER DINNER OPTIONS: Same as Day One
DESSERT: "A" and/or "Neutral" foods

<u>Snacks From Dinner To Bedtime:</u>
Choose anything from "Neutral", or continue with "A" fruits and/or nuts and raisins.

DAY THREE

BREAKFAST: Same as Day One

LUNCH:

Chicken Thighs with Vegetables*   4 servings

8 pieces chicken
1/4 cup grated Parmesan cheese
2 tablespoons butter
4 tablespoons butter, melted
1 cup grated carrots
1 cup broccoli, chopped
1 onion, chopped
Salt to taste
Pepper to taste
Oregano to taste

1. Preheat oven to 350°F. Place chicken on a baking sheet. Sprinkle the chicken with butter and Parmesan cheese. Bake until chicken is tender. Approximately 45 minutes.
2. In a frying pan, melt butter over medium-high heat. Add carrots, broccoli, and onion and cook, tossing often, for 5 minutes, until broccoli is cooked but still crisp.
3. Serve chicken mixed in with vegetables.

COMPATIBLE with "B" and "Neutral" foods
*Optional for Working People: Same as Day One or Fried Chicken. (See A&B Cookbook.)

DINNER:

Pasta Parisian   4-6 servings

1 pound rigatoni (or other pasta)
1 large eggplant
1 cup ricotta cheese or cottage cheese
1/2 cup heavy cream, diluted with water
1/2 cup olive oil
2 large cloves garlic, crushed through a press
2 carrots, cut into thin strips, about 3 inches long
2 celery stalks, cut into thin strips, about 3 inches long
4 onions, finely chopped
Soy sauce to taste
1 teaspoon oregano
1 teaspoon basil
Cayenne pepper to taste

1. Cut eggplant into 3/4-inch cubes. Put eggplant in a strainer. Sprinkle sufficient salt over eggplant. Let stand until fluid drains off, 45 minutes.
2. In a saucepan, cook pasta in boiling salted water until tender but firm. Remove from heat and drain.
3. In a deep frying pan (a wok is preferred), cook onions and garlic in hot oil until brown. Add 3/4-inch eggplant. Season with soy sauce, oregano, basil, and cayenne pepper. Reduce heat, cook, stirring occasionally, at least 1/2 hour. Add ricotta or cottage cheese and 1/2 cup heavy cream. Add mixture to rigatoni. Mix well.

COMPATIBLE with "A" and "Neutral" foods
OTHER DINNER OPTIONS: Same as Day One
DESSERT: Same as Day One

DAY FOUR

BREAKFAST: Same as Day One

LUNCH:

Cauliflower Soufflé Côte d'Azur*　　　　4 servings

1 large cauliflower, cored and broken into small florets
3 tablespoons oil
2 egg yolks
1/4 cup parsley, chopped
1 pinch sweet Hungarian (or regular) paprika
1 pinch nutmeg

1. Preheat oven to 350°F.
2. In a saucepan, cook cauliflower in boiling salted water until just tender, about 10 minutes. Remove from heat.
3. In a small soufflé dish, heat oil.
4. Whisk two egg yolks with 3 tablespoons oil, nutmeg, pepper, and parsley.
5. Spread mixture over cauliflower. Bake until soufflé is golden brown, about 10–15 minutes.

COMPATIBLE with "A", "B", and "Neutral" foods
*Optional for Working People: Same as Day One

Note: Cauliflower contains pantothenic acid which detoxifies cells and plays a vital role in the biochemical reactions within the body—and it enhances production of healthy skin.

DINNER:

A&B Power Salad (Same as Day One)

VARIATION: Potatoes may be added to the A&B Power Salad for a different texture.

1. In a vegetable steamer, place unpeeled potatoes over boiling water for 20 minutes.
2. Cook until tender.
3. Remove from heat. Place potatoes in a large bowl. Let stand until potatoes are cool enough to handle. Peel.
4. Cut potatoes into 1/4-inch slices or dice into small cubes. Add potatoes, mayonnaise, or dip/dressing to the A&B Power Salad. Mix well.

COMPATIBLE with "A", "B", or "Neutral" foods
OTHER DINNER OPTIONS: Same as Day One
DESSERT: Same as Day One

DAY FIVE

BREAKFAST: Same as Day One

LUNCH:

Cabbage Budapest*   2–3 servings

1 white cabbage, sliced
1 pound onions, diced
2 cups vegetable broth (or 2 cups water/2 bouillon cubes)
2 cups heavy cream
2 tablespoons butter
1 cup sour cream
Sea salt to taste
2 teaspoons Hungarian (or regular) paprika
Soy sauce to taste

1. In a large saucepan, sauté onions in butter until golden brown. Add vegetable broth or bouillon.
2. Place cabbage in saucepan and cook for 15–20 minutes. Remove from heat and drain cabbage.
3. Combine heavy cream with paprika and season to taste. Sprinkle mixture over cabbage. Let stand 10 minutes.

COMPATIBLE with "A", "B", and "Neutral" foods
*Optional for Working People: Same as Day One

DINNER:

Roast Chicken Hawaii   4-6 servings

1 whole chicken, about 3 pounds
2 tablespoons butter
2 tablespoons olive oil
Pineapples, diced
1 teaspoon dried thyme
Salt and pepper to taste
1 cup dry white wine

1. Preheat oven to 350°F. Season chicken inside and out with sea salt and pepper. Place 1/2 teaspoon thyme in cavity. Tie legs together and rub butter over skin. Place in a large roasting pan with water.
2. Roast chicken for 15 minutes. Arrange diced pineapples around chicken. Sprinkle remaining thyme over chicken. Pour dry white wine over all and bake 1 hour and 15 minutes. Add water when wine evaporates.

COMPATIBLE with "B" and "Neutral" foods
OTHER DINNER OPTIONS: Same as Day One
DESSERT: "B" and/or "Neutral"

DAY SIX

BREAKFAST: Same as Day One

LUNCH:

Waldorf Astoria Salad*

2 cups diced apples (about 2 medium apples)
2 sweet seedless oranges, diced
1/2 pound cooked chicken, diced (good use of leftovers)
1 cup celery, coarsely chopped
1 cup mayonnaise
1 cup sour cream
4 tablespoons heavy cream, whipped
1/2 cup coarsely chopped walnuts
1 dash cognac
2 tablespoons lemon juice or vinegar
1 dash salt

In a medium bowl, combine all ingredients, except whipped cream, sour cream, and walnuts. Mix well. Chill thoroughly. Add whipped cream, sour cream, and walnuts before serving. Serve on lettuce. Leftovers should be refrigerated and can be taken to work next day.

COMPATIBLE with "B" and "Neutral" foods
*Optional for Working People: Same as Day One

DINNER:

A&B Power Salad (Same as Day One)

OTHER DINNER OPTIONS: Same as Day One
DESSERT: Same as Day One

DAY SEVEN

BREAKFAST: Same as Day One
LUNCH:

Mozzarella with Tomatoes *   2 servings

2 large tomatoes, sliced
1 ball of fresh mozzarella, sliced
Fresh basil
Vinegar
Olive oil
Salt
Pepper

1. Cut tomatoes and mozzarella in thin slices. Arrange on a plate.
2. In a small bowl, combine vinegar and oil. Pour mixture over mozzarella and tomatoes. Add salt and pepper to taste. Garnish with fresh basil.

COMPATIBLE with "A", "B", and "Neutral" foods
*Optional for Working People: Same as Day One—or leftover Waldorf Astoria Salad from Day Six

DINNER:

Eggplant Normandy   4 servings

2 large eggplants (or 4 small)
6 cloves garlic, crushed through a press
4 small onions, peeled
2 medium tomatoes, pureed
2 cups olive oil
1 bunch parsley, chopped
1 bunch cilantro, chopped
Salt
Pepper
Celery salt

217

1. Preheat oven to 300°F.
2. With a sharp knife, remove stem head of eggplants. Cut eggplants into 1/2-inch slices.
3. Chop cilantro and parsley. Puree tomatoes. Add garlic. Mix well.
4. In a large frying pan, heat cooking oil. Place eggplants in oil. Fry until brown.
5. On a baking sheet, place eggplant slices. Sprinkle tomato-cilantro-parsley mixture over eggplants. Bake for 20 minutes, until crispy. Season to taste.

COMPATIBLE with "B" and "Neutral" foods (if eaten without tomatoes, also compatible with "A")
OTHER DINNER OPTIONS: Same as Day One
DESSERT: Neutral or "A" or "B"

DAY EIGHT

BREAKFAST: Same as Day One

LUNCH:

Rochelle's Meatballs*   4 servings

2 pounds ground meat
2 onions, chopped
2 onions, sliced
2 stalks celery, chopped
3–4 cloves garlic
1/2 bunch parsley
1 large can Italian peeled tomatoes, 12 ounces
Olive oil to taste
Soy flour as needed, see below
Soy sauce to taste
Sea salt to taste
Pepper to taste
Celery salt, oregano, basil to taste

1. In a food processor or blender combine chopped onions, celery, garlic, parsley, sea salt, pepper, celery salt, oregano and basil. Process vegetables. Process until a puree forms.
2. Mix vegetable puree into chop meat; mix very well; add soy flour until it is still moist but can be formed into balls by rolling mixture into 1 1/2" diameter balls in palms of hands.
3. In a frying pan, combine butter and sliced onions until lightly brown. Add salt, pepper, oregano, parsley, celery salt, and basil. Mix well. Add Italian peeled tomatoes. Chop up while cooking. Add meatballs and cook (low), turning, about 1 hour. Add soy sauce to taste.

COMPATIBLE with "B" and "Neutral" foods
*Optional for Working People: Same as Day One or leftover salads

DINNER:

Creamy Cauliflower Soup   4 servings

6 cups spring water
2 medium cauliflowers, cored and coarsely chopped
1 onion, chopped
1 clove garlic, crushed through a press
2 tablespoons butter
1 tablespoon olive oil
2 stalks celery, chopped
8 scallions, chopped
2 tablespoons vegetable broth (or water and bouillon cube)
1/8 teaspoon fresh ground black pepper
1/8 teaspoon nutmeg
1 teaspoon dried basil
1/2 teaspoon dried thyme
1 teaspoon dried marjoram
1/2 teaspoon celery or sea salt

In a large saucepan, melt butter and heat oil. Add scallions, onions, garlic, cauliflower and celery. Season with salt and pepper to taste. Cook over medium heat for several minutes, stirring frequently. Add vegetable broth or the water and bouillon; bring to a boil. Add basil, thyme, marjoram. Simmer, covered, over low heat until cauliflower is tender, for 10–15 minutes. Remove cover and cool slightly. In blender, process until soup is smooth and creamy. Add nutmeg to taste.

COMPATIBLE with "A", "B", and "Neutral" foods
OTHER DINNER OPTIONS: Same as Day One or any other Dinner choice
DESSERT: Neutral, or "A" or "B"

DAY NINE

BREAKFAST: Same as Day One

LUNCH:

Mushrooms Lyon*   2–3 servings

1/2 pound mushrooms
2 tablespoons butter
1 tablespoon fresh lemon juice
Dash sea salt
Dash garlic powder
Soy sauce

1. Wash mushrooms; cut and discard ends from stems. Cut mushrooms into slices.
2. In a saucepan, melt butter. Add mushrooms, tossing lightly in butter, until soft. Add lemon juice. Season to taste.

COMPATIBLE with "A", "B", and "Neutral" foods
*Optional for Working People: Same as Day One

DINNER:

Spaghetti à la Toscana   4 servings

1 pound spaghetti
4 onions, chopped
2 large cloves garlic, crushed through a press
1 1/2 pounds mushrooms, sliced
2 tablespoons butter
1/2 pound grated fresh cheese (above 60% fat)
1 cup heavy cream
1 teaspoon fresh basil, chopped
1 pinch salt
1 pinch pepper
1 teaspoon basil
1 teaspoon oregano

1. In a medium saucepan, cook onions and mushrooms in butter until softened but not brown. Add garlic, salt, and pepper to taste. Add fresh cheese. Stir until melted. Add cream. Mix well; set aside.
2. In a large pasta pot, cook pasta in boiling salted water until tender but firm. Remove from heat and drain. Sprinkle mixture over spaghetti. Sprinkle fresh basil and oregano to taste.

COMPATIBLE with "A" and "Neutral" foods
OTHER DINNER OPTIONS: Same as Day One
DESSERT: Same as Day One

DAY TEN

BREAKFAST: Same as Day One

LUNCH:

Zurich "Geschnetzeltes"*   4 servings

1 1/2 pounds beef or veal
1 pound mushrooms, sliced
1 can or frozen green peas
1 cup heavy cream
2 large onions, chopped
4 cloves garlic, crushed through a press
Celery salt to taste
Garlic powder to taste
Salt and pepper to taste

1. Cut meat in 1/2-inch slices with a sharp knife or have the butcher prepare it. Season with celery salt and pepper.
2. In a small frying pan, combine butter, onions, and garlic. Heat until lightly brown. Add meat and cook, turning, until brown. Reduce heat and add mushrooms, seasoning, and heavy cream. Simmer, stirring occasionally, about 1 hour. Add peas and season to taste.

COMPATIBLE with "B" and "Neutral" foods
*Optional for Working People: Same as Day One or any leftovers

DINNER:

Potato Salad d'Alsace   4 servings

6 new potatoes, unpeeled
Beef salami, diced into cubes (optional: smoked fish), quantity to taste
1 fresh cucumber, sliced
1 large tomato, cut into small cubes
2 large pickles (sour or sweet dill), chopped into very thin slices
1/2 bunch chives, chopped
Scallions, to taste, chopped
1 onion, chopped
Mayonnaise and/or chunky Blue Cheese dressing, to taste
Olive or any other natural oil to taste
Vinegar to taste
Salt, pepper, and celery salt to taste

1. In a vegetable steamer, place potatoes over boiling water for 20 to 30 minutes until just tender. Remove from heat. Place potatoes in a large bowl. Let stand until potatoes are cool enough to handle. Peel potatoes. Cut potatoes into 1/2-inch cubes.
2. Add oil, vinegar, vegetables, cucumber, salami (or fish), and mayonnaise to potatoes. Mix well, but gently.
3. Eat hot or cold.

COMPATIBLE with "A" and "Neutral" foods
OTHER DINNER OPTIONS: Same as Day One or leftovers
DESSERT: Same as Day One

DAY ELEVEN

BREAKFAST: Same as Day One

LUNCH:

<u>A&B Power Salad</u>* (Same as Day One)

COMPATIBLE with Neutral, "A", or "B"
*Optional for Working People: Same as Day One

DINNER:

DON'T FORGET TO PREPARE ALL BEAN DINNERS AHEAD OF TIME:
Soaking beans requires at least 3 to 4 hours and cooking time, a low simmer of 4 to 5 hours!

<u>Ramses Beans & Ramses Salad</u>

Old Egyptian recipe; beans should be eaten with Ramses Salad to ensure proper digestion.
VARIATION: add chopped onions, dressed with vinegar, pepper, sea salt, and cumin.

2 pounds small fava beans
1 pound skinless fava beans (found in Oriental groceries)
1 pound Garbanzo beans (chickpeas)
1/2 pound yellow lentils
1 large bulb of garlic, crushed through a press
2 tablespoons cumin
2 tablespoons dried coriander
Salt to taste
Pepper to taste

1. Wash beans and lentils separately. In a big bowl, put fava beans, skinless fava beans, and Garbanzo beans. Cover beans with plenty of cold spring water. Soak beans for at least 3–4 hours. Remove from water.
2. In a large pot add fava beans and Garbanzo beans. Cover with water to 4 inches above beans. Bring to a boil, then reduce heat.
3. Simmer over medium-low heat for 4-5 hours, until soft. Check the water levels every hour, adding water if necessary.
4. Add lentils during last hour.
5. Add garlic, cumin, coriander, sea salt, and pepper. Let stand for 30 minutes. Serve warm. Top the Ramses Beans with Ramses Salad.

VARIATION: mash beans with mixer and top it with Ramses Salad).

COMPATIBLE with "A", "B", and "Neutral" foods
DESSERT: Neutral, "A" or "B"

HELPFUL TIP: *Leftovers can be stored in freezer. Put small portions in bowls or plastic bags for work lunches or other dinners.*

Ramses Salad

5–6 fresh hot peppers, such as jalapenos
2–3 large tomatoes
1 head of lettuce
6 large cloves of garlic
2 large onions
1 tablespoon coriander
1 bunch cilantro
1 tablespoon cumin
Salt and pepper to taste
1/2 cup vinegar
1/2 cup olive oil

In a food processor, combine all ingredients. Process until well blended to form a pulp. Top Ramses Beans with 3 tablespoons Ramses Salad.

HELPFUL TIP: *In a jar, put remaining Ramses Salad. Cover with olive oil, 2-inches above pulp. Refrigerate for later use. Without bread for lunch; with whole wheat bread or pita for dinner.*

DAY TWELVE

BREAKFAST: Same as Day One

LUNCH:

Fettuccine Alfredo*   2-3 servings

1 pound fettuccine
8 tablespoons butter, softened
1/4 cup heavy cream
1 cup grated mozzarella cheese
Freshly ground pepper

1. Cook pasta in boiling salted water until tender but firm. Remove from heat and drain.
2. Place fettuccine in a warm bowl or on a serving platter. Add butter, cream, and half the mozzarella cheese. Toss fettuccine noodles gently until they are evenly coated. Serve immediately, topped with pepper and remaining mozzarella cheese.

COMPATIBLE with "A" and "Neutral" foods
*Optional for Working People: Same as Day One or bring leftover salads

DINNER:

Baked Sole with Oranges   4 servings

1 1/2 pounds sole fillets
1/2 teaspoon salt
1/4 teaspoon pepper
1 teaspoon soy flour
1/4 cup fresh orange juice
1/4 cup fresh lemon juice
1 whole orange

1. Preheat oven to 425°F.
2. Arrange fish in a baking dish large enough to hold fillets flat in a single layer. Season with salt and pepper. Add orange juice and lemon juice. Cover and refrigerate 1 hour.
3. Use a serrated knife to cut away peel from orange. Cut between membranes to remove whole sections. Place in a small bowl and set aside.
4. Remove fish from refrigerator and cover dish tightly with aluminum foil. Bake 8–10 minutes, until firm and opaque throughout.
5. Transfer fillets to serving plate. Pour cooking liquid into a small saucepan.
6. Dissolve soy flour in 2 tablespoons cold water. Stir into liquid in saucepan and bring to a boil over medium-high heat; stirring until thickened. Spread sauce over fillets; garnish with orange slices.

COMPATIBLE with "B" and "Neutral" foods
OTHER DINNER OPTIONS: Same as Day One
DESSERT: "B" and "Neutral"

DAY THIRTEEN

BREAKFAST: Same as Day One

LUNCH:

Chef Salad*

Lettuce (quantity to taste)
Tomatoes, sliced or diced into cubes
Cucumbers, thinly sliced
Broccoli, sliced
Cauliflower, sliced
Carrots, thinly sliced
Onions, sliced or diced into cubes
1–2 boiled eggs, sliced
Swiss cheese, thinly sliced
Smoked ham, sliced
Cooked turkey or chicken, rectangular slices
Oil to taste
Vinegar to taste
Salt to taste
Pepper to taste
Mayonnaise (OPTIONAL: dip or salad dressing)

Cut vegetables. In a large bowl, combine all vegetables, smoked and/or cooked ham, cooked turkey, or chicken. Add oil, vinegar, salt, and pepper. Add mayonnaise, dip, or dressing.

COMPATIBLE with "B" and "Neutral" foods
*Optional for Working People: Same as Day One or bring in leftovers

DINNER:

Mozzarella Pizza

A&B Pizza Dough and A&B Pizza Sauce
(Same as Day One; also see A&B Cookbook)
3 cups shredded mozzarella cheese (about 12 ounces)
2 tablespoons pine nuts

1. Prepare pizza dough.
2. Prepare pizza sauce.
3. Preheat oven to 350°F.
4. Spread pizza sauce evenly over dough. Top with mozzarella and pine nuts. Place baking sheet on lowest shelf in oven (or the floor of a gas oven). Bake until crust is firm and golden brown. Serve warm.

COMPATIBLE with "A" and "Neutral" foods
OTHER DINNER OPTIONS: Same as Day One
DESSERT: Same as Day One

DAY FOURTEEN

BREAKFAST: Same as Day One

LUNCH:

Cabbage Budapest* (See Day Five Lunch)

COMPATIBLE with "A", "B", and "Neutral" foods
*Optional for Working People: Same as Day One

DINNER:

Austrian Baked Potatoes "Arnold"   4 servings

4 large potatoes, unpeeled
Butter, 1 tablespoon for each potato
Sour cream or ready-to-buy fresh creamy Italian garlic dip or fresh sour cream dip without preservatives
Herbs, parsley, and chives
Sea salt
Pepper
Aluminum foil

1. With a sharp knife, make a lengthwise cut across each potato. Season potatoes with salt and pepper to taste. Top each potato with a tablespoon of butter. Wrap each potato in aluminum foil.
2. Preheat oven to 400°F. Place potatoes on baking sheet. Bake until tender, about 45 minutes to 1 hour.
3. In a bowl, mix sour cream with parsley and chives to taste.
4. Serve hot; in or out of aluminum foil.
5. Garnish with herbed sour cream.

COMPATIBLE with "A" and "Neutral" foods
OTHER DINNER OPTIONS: Same as Day One
DESSERT: Same as Day One

DAY FIFTEEN

BREAKFAST: Same as Day One
LUNCH:

Mozzarella with Tomatoes*   2 servings

2 large tomatoes, sliced
1 ball of fresh mozzarella, sliced
Fresh basil
Vinegar to taste
Olive oil to taste
Salt to taste
Pepper to taste

1. Cut tomatoes and mozzarella in thin slices. Arrange on a plate.
2. In a small bowl, combine vinegar and oil. Pour mixture over mozzarella and tomatoes. Add salt and pepper to taste. Garnish with fresh basil.

COMPATIBLE with "A", "B", and "Neutral" foods
*Optional for Working People: Same as Day One

DINNER:

Italian Stuffed Green Peppers   4 servings

2 pounds ground meat
2 middle-size onions, sliced
2 middle-size onions, cut in halves
8 green peppers (or 8 zucchini or 8 large tomatoes)
5 cloves garlic, crushed through a press (or garlic powder to taste)
1/2 bunch parsley, chopped
1/2 bunch cilantro, chopped
1/2 bunch dill, chopped
2 tablespoons butter or olive oil
1 bouillon cube
Pinch saffron
Juice of 1 lemon

1. In a food processor or blender, combine parsley, cilantro, garlic, and dill with a small amount of water. Process until a puree forms.
2. In a large bowl, combine meat, eggs, vegetable puree, and seasonings (except saffron and lemon). Blend well.
3. With a sharp knife, cut off tops of green peppers. Carefully remove seeds and veins, leaving stems intact.
4. Stuff vegetable with meat mixture.
5. Preheat oven to 350°F. Place stuffed peppers in a large greased baking dish. Bake for 45 minutes to 1 hour.
6. In a small frying pan, heat 1 cup of water and add 1 bouillon cube, saffron and lemon juice. Add baking dish. Bake until peppers are tender. Remove from oven.
7. Top with sour cream. Serve warm.

COMPATIBLE with "B" and "Neutral" foods
OTHER DINNER OPTIONS: Same as Day One
DESSERT: "B" and Neutral

DAY SIXTEEN

BREAKFAST: Same as Day One
LUNCH:

Sylvia's Tuna Salad*   2 servings

1 (6 1/2 ounce) can tuna, in oil or water
1/4 cup capers, either small capers or large cut in half
3 tablespoons chopped onions
2 tablespoons mustard
1/2 cup pickles, diced
1/3 cup parsley, chopped
Olive oil, quantity to taste
1 teaspoon fresh lemon juice (or vinegar)
1/4 teaspoon pepper
Salt to taste
Garlic salt to taste

In a medium bowl, drain then mash tuna with oil and mustard. Add onions, lemon juice, pickles, ½ the capers, sea salt, and pepper. Mix well. Serve on lettuce. Garnish with remaining capers or pickle slices.

COMPATIBLE with "B" and "Neutral" foods
*Optional for Working People: Same as Day One

DINNER:

A&B Power Salad
(Same as Day One with anything from the "Neutral", "A", or "B" groups)

OTHER DINNER OPTIONS: Same as Day One
DESSERT: Same as Day One

DAY SEVENTEEN

BREAKFAST: Same as Day One
LUNCH:

Macaroni & Cheese*   4 servings

1/2 pound macaroni; any variety
3 cups shredded mozzarella
4–5 cloves garlic, crushed through a press
1 teaspoon oregano
1 teaspoon thyme

1. In a large saucepan, cook macaroni in boiling salted water until tender but firm. Remove from heat and drain.
2. Combine mozzarella with oregano, thyme, and garlic. Sprinkle mixture over macaroni.
3. Preheat oven to 300°F. Place macaroni in a greased baking dish. Bake until macaroni is golden brown and crisp, 20 minutes.

COMPATIBLE with "A" and "Neutral" foods
*Optional for Working People: Same as Day One

DINNER:

Crispy Rice Balls St. Tropez   4-6 servings

1 cup brown rice
1 1/2 tablespoons butter
1/4 cup olive oil
4 cups chicken broth (or 4 bouillon cubes, dissolved in 4 cups water)
Wheat or soy flour
Bread crumbs
3 egg yolks
1/4 pound finely shredded mozzarella cheese
1/4 cup feta cheese
1 tablespoon parsley, minced
1/8 tablespoon freshly ground pepper
1/4 teaspoon grated nutmeg

235

1. Prepare rice (basic recipe). Let cool.
2. In a large bowl, beat 1 egg yolk. Add rice along with cheese, parsley, pepper, nutmeg. Blend well. Cover mixture and refrigerate at least 1 hour, until chilled.
3. In a small bowl, beat 2 egg yolks with 2 teaspoons water; set aside.
4. Scoop mixture. Shape rice with the palms of your hands into balls (1 1/2 inches).
5. First roll rice balls in flour; then egg yolk; then breadcrumbs. Cover with plastic wrap. Refrigerate for 2 hours.
6. In a heavy frying pan heat 3 inches of oil to 375°F. Place chilled rice balls in hot oil. Fry, occasionally turning, for 3–5 minutes, until golden brown. Remove with a spoon. Drain on paper towels. Serve at once.

COMPATIBLE with "A" and "Neutral" foods
OTHER DINNER OPTIONS: Same as Day One
DESSERT: Same as Day One

DAY EIGHTEEN

BREAKFAST: Same as Day One

LUNCH:

Smoked Salmon and Cheese*   4 servings

3 ounces thinly sliced smoked salmon
1/4 teaspoon hot pepper sauce
Dash of lemon juice
8 ounces cream cheese, softened
1 cup fresh dill or parsley
3/4 cup grated Parmesan or feta cheese (about 3 ounces)

1. Preheat oven to 400°F. In a small bowl or food processor, combine cream cheese, Parmesan or feta cheese, lemon juice, and hot sauce. Blend well.

2. Cut smoked salmon into about 30 pieces. Spoon about 2 teaspoons of cheese mixture over pieces of salmon and top each with dill or parsley. Bake until cheese is softened, about 5 minutes. Serve warm.

COMPATIBLE with "B" and "Neutral" foods
*Optional for Working People: Same as Day One

DINNER:

Pizza Athena

A&B Pizza Dough (see basic recipe, same as Day One or cookbook)
A&B Pizza Sauce (see basic recipe, same as Day One or cookbook)
1 1/2 cups feta, crumbled
Olives (quantity to taste)
3 cups mozzarella, shredded

1. Prepare pizza dough.
2. Prepare pizza sauce.
3. Preheat oven to 350°F
4. Spread sauce evenly over dough. Top with feta, mozzarella, and olives.
5. Place baking sheet on lowest shelf in oven and bake until crust is firm and golden brown, 15 to 20 minutes.

COMPATIBLE with "A" and "Neutral" foods
OTHER DINNER OPTIONS: Same as Day One
DESSERT: Same as Day One

DAY NINETEEN

BREAKFAST: Same as Day One

LUNCH:

Cauliflower Soufflé Côte d'Azur*　　　4 servings

1 large cauliflower (cored and cut into small florets)
3 tablespoons olive oil
2 egg yolks
1/2 cup parsley, chopped
1 pinch sweet Hungarian (or regular) paprika
1 pinch nutmeg

1. Preheat oven to 350°F.
2. In a large saucepan, cook cauliflower in boiling salted water for 10 minutes. Remove from heat.
3. In a small soufflé dish, heat oil. Then put cauliflower in dish.
4. Whisk two egg yolks, with 3 teaspoons oil, nutmeg, pepper, and parsley in separate bowl.
5. Spread egg mixture over cauliflower. Bake until soufflé is golden brown, about 10 minutes.

COMPATIBLE with "A", "B", and "Neutral" foods
*Optional for Working People: Same as Day One

DINNER:

Classic Roast Chicken　　　4 servings

1 whole chicken
1 medium onion, quartered
1 medium onion, sliced
2 carrots, thickly sliced
2 zucchini, sliced
2 tablespoons butter
2 tablespoons olive oil
1 tablespoon soy flour
1 cup chicken stock or water with chicken bouillon cube

1 tablespoon dried thyme
Salt and pepper to taste

1. Rinse and dry the chicken.
2. Preheat oven to 350°F. Season chicken liberally with salt and pepper inside and out. Put small quartered onions and thyme inside cavity and tie legs together. Rub butter all over chicken.
3. Put oil in a large oval gratin dish or shallow roasting pan. Scatter sliced onions, zucchini, and carrots around the dish. Place chicken on top.
4. Roast chicken in oven until it is golden brown, about 25 minutes per pound.
5. Remove chicken to a serving platter and cover with foil to keep warm.
6. Remove all but 2 tablespoons fat from pan. Place over medium heat, add soy flour, and cook, stirring, until thickened. Season with salt and pepper to taste. Strain into a gravy boat and serve with chicken.

COMPATIBLE with "B" and "Neutral" foods
OTHER DINNER OPTIONS: Same as Day One
DESSERT: "B" and "Neutral"

DAY TWENTY

BREAKFAST: Same as Day One
LUNCH:

Hawaiian Chicken Salad*   4 servings

1/2 pound cooked chicken (leftovers), diced
2 cups pineapple, diced
1 cup mayonnaise
Dash vinegar
Dash pepper
Pinch garlic salt
Pinch nutmeg

1. In a medium bowl, combine all ingredients; mix well.
2. Chill thoroughly. Serve on lettuce; top with diced pineapples.

COMPATIBLE with "B" and "Neutral" foods
*Optional for Working People: Same as Day One

DINNER:

Potato Salzburg with Sour Cream   4 servings

10 medium-sized new potatoes
1/2 cup sour cream
1/2 bunch chives, minced

1. Preheat oven to 400°F.
2. Arrange potatoes on a baking sheet. Bake potatoes until tender. Place potatoes in a large bowl. Let stand until potatoes are cool enough to handle.
3. Halve potatoes. Scoop out a little bit of potato and fill cavity with 2 teaspoons sour cream.
4. Cook until heated through, about 10 minutes. Garnish with chives

COMPATIBLE with "A" and "Neutral" foods
OTHER DINNER OPTIONS: Same as Day One
DESSERT: Same as Day One

DAY TWENTY-ONE

BREAKFAST: Same as Day One
LUNCH:

<u>A&B Power Salad*</u> (Same as Day One)
COMPATIBLE with anything from the "Neutral", "A",
or, "B" groups.
*Optional for Working People: Same as Day One

DINNER:

<u>Oriental Lentil Soup</u>   4-6 servings

1 1/2 cups lentils (already soaked for 3-4 hours)
2 cups vegetable or chicken bouillon (cubes in 2 cups water)
8 cups spring water
1 large onion, minced
1 clove garlic, crushed through a press
2 stalks celery, chopped
2 large carrots, chopped
2 tablespoons fresh parsley, chopped
1/2 teaspoon sea salt
1 teaspoon dried oregano
1 teaspoon sweet Hungarian (or regular) paprika
1/2 teaspoon dried thyme
3 tablespoons olive oil

1. In a saucepan, melt oil over medium-high heat. Add onions,
    tossing for 5 minutes until crisp-tender.
2. Add garlic, carrots, and celery. Add seasonings and herbs; mix
    well, tossing for 3–4 minutes. Add vegetable or chicken
    bouillon; cook for 3 minutes.
3. Add lentils and 8 cups hot water. Simmer over low heat for 60
    minutes.

COMPATIBLE with "A", "B", and "Neutral" foods
OTHER DINNER OPTIONS: Same as Day One
DESSERT: Same as Day One

DAY TWENTY-TWO

BREAKFAST: Same as Day One
LUNCH:

Broccoli Milanese*   2 servings

4 stalks broccoli, washed with stems cut off
2 tablespoons butter
2 tablespoons fresh lemon juice
Seasoning to taste

1. Cut broccoli into individual florets. Place in covered vegetable steamer over boiling water until tender, for 7 minutes
2. In a small saucepan, melt butter; mix with lemon juice. Pour sauce over hot broccoli. Season to taste.

COMPATIBLE with "A", "B", and "Neutral" foods
*Optional for Working People: Same as Day One

DINNER:

Swordfish Steak   2-4 servings

4 swordfish steaks, 4–6 ounces each
2 tablespoons grated Parmesan cheese
2 cloves garlic, peeled
1/3 cup olive oil
1/4 cup pine nuts
1 cup fresh basil leaves
1/4 teaspoon salt
1/8 teaspoon pepper
Lemon slices

1. Preheat oven to 425°F. Arrange fish steaks in a large, lightly oiled baking dish. In a food processor, combine basil, garlic, pine nuts, Parmesan cheese, salt, and pepper. Puree until smooth. With machine on, slowly pour in olive oil. Process until mixture is well blended.

2. Spread mixture evenly over swordfish steaks. Cover dish loosely with aluminum foil. Bake until steaks are white throughout but still moist, 10–12 minutes. Garnish with thin slices of lemon.

COMPATIBLE with "B" and "Neutral" foods
OTHER DINNER OPTIONS: Same as Day One
DESSERT: Same as Day One

DAY TWENTY-THREE

BREAKFAST: Same as Day One
LUNCH:

Asparagus Salad*   3-4 servings

1 head lettuce
1/2 head red leaf lettuce
1/2 pound fresh (or canned) asparagus
3 tablespoons olive oil
1 tablespoon vinegar
1 clove garlic, crushed through a press
1/2 tablespoon mustard
Sea salt to taste
Fresh ground black pepper

1. Wash salad; dry and break into pieces. Cut off and discard heavy ends from asparagus.
2. In a medium saucepan, cook asparagus in boiling salted water until tender, 3–5 minutes. Remove from water, drain well, and cut into 1 1/2-inch pieces. Combine with lettuce.
3. For dressing; combine oil, mustard, sea salt, and lemon juice (or vinegar) in cup. Add pepper to taste. Mix well. Pour over salad.

COMPATIBLE with "A", "B", and "Neutral" foods
*Optional for Working People: Same as Day One

DINNER:

French Cabbage Roll   4 servings

1 large white cabbage
2 pounds ground meat
1/2 pound mushrooms (optional)
2 whole eggs
1/2 cup sour cream
3 large onions, chopped
1 clove garlic, crushed through a press
4 tablespoons butter or olive oil
1 pinch thyme
1 pinch cumin
1 pinch fennel seed
1 pinch pepper
1 pinch sweet Hungarian (or regular) paprika
1 pinch sea salt

1. Place cabbage in a vegetable steamer (or in boiling water) until leaves are tender when pierced with tip of sharp knife. Separate tender leaves.
2. In a small frying pan, cook onions until golden brown.
3. In a big bowl, combine ground meat, onions, eggs, and spices. Mix well.
4. On a big plate, arrange leaves and form meat mixture into balls. Arrange meat mixture on cabbage leaves. Wrap cabbage around meat. Bind with cotton string or thread.
5. In a large frying pan, melt 4 tablespoons of butter over medium heat. Add onions and cabbage rolls. Cook cabbage rolls, turning, until brown. When golden brown, add sour cream and 1/2 cup of water. Cook on low for 45 minutes. Serve warm.

COMPATIBLE with "B" and "Neutral" foods
OTHER DINNER OPTIONS: Same as Day One
DESSERT: "B" and "Neutral" foods.

DAY TWENTY-FOUR

BREAKFAST: Same as Day One
LUNCH:

Swiss Cheese Salad*   2-3 servings

1/2 pound Swiss cheese, cut in thin 1/2-inch strips
2 medium onions, thinly sliced into rings
Olive oil to taste; vinegar to taste
Salt to taste; pepper to taste

In a medium bowl, combine all ingredients. Add salt and pepper to taste.
Mix well.

COMPATIBLE with "B" and "Neutral" foods
*Optional for Working People: Same as Day One

DINNER:

Pasta di Paesano   4 servings

1/2 pound elbow macaroni
Crumbled feta cheese (quantity to taste)
1 cup heavy cream
4 cloves garlic, crushed through a press
Fresh mint (quantity to taste), chopped
Fresh spinach (quantity to taste), chopped
Olive oil to taste

1. Combine fresh spinach, fresh mint, feta cheese, cream, olive oil
    and garlic; simmer on low.
2. In a saucepan, cook macaroni in boiling salted water until tender
    but firm. Remove from heat and drain. Add cream mixture to
    macaroni. Mix well.

COMPATIBLE with "A" and "Neutral" foods
OTHER DINNER OPTIONS: Same as Day One
DESSERT: Same as Day One

DAY TWENTY-FIVE

BREAKFAST: Same as Day One

LUNCH:

Artichokes Venetian*   2 servings

4 artichokes
Several stalks celery
1 bay leaf
1 clove garlic, crushed through a press

1. Wash artichokes. Trim end of stems. Snip thorny tip off each
    leaf.
2. In a vegetable steamer, place artichokes, garlic, celery stalks,
    and bay leaf, over boiling water; steam for 30 to 40 minutes. As
    soon as leaves can be easily removed, discard bay leaf, celery
    and garlic. Serve with melted butter for dipping.

COMPATIBLE with "A", "B", and "Neutral" foods
*Optional for Working People: Same as Day One

DINNER:

Ramses Beans & Ramses Salad
(Same as Day Eleven)

**REMEMBER TO PLAN AHEAD: Soaking beans
requires at least 3 to 4 hours plus 4 to 5 hours of
cooking time!**

COMPATIBLE: "A", "B", and "Neutral" foods
OTHER DINNER OPTIONS: Same as Day One
DESSERT: Same as Day One

DAY TWENTY-SIX

BREAKFAST: Same as Day One

LUNCH:

<u>A&B Power Salad*</u> (Same as Day One)

COMPATIBLE with anything from the "Neutral", "A", or "B" groups
*Optional for Working People: Same as Day One

<u>BBQ Grilled Meat and Veggies</u>

1 large flank steak or 2 small steaks of choice-or-1 lb. Italian sausage-or-
1 lb. chopped meat for hamburgers
2 large ripe tomatoes
1 large onion
1 eggplant
1 zucchini
Seasoning to taste

1. Cut tomatoes, onions, eggplants and zucchini into ¼" slices; baste with olive oil on both sides and set aside.
2. Preheat barbeque and when hot, put meat of choice on grill and cook as normal.
3. When meat is half done; take vegetables and put directly on grill. Turning once.
4. Serve meat and vegetables topped with condiments and seasoning to taste.

COMPATIBLE with "B" and "Neutral" foods
OTHER DINNER OPTIONS: Same as Day One
DESSERT: Same as Day One

DAY TWENTY-SEVEN

BREAKFAST: Same as Day One

LUNCH:

Classic Potato Soup   4-6 servings

8 peeled potatoes (medium to large), chopped in cubes
6–7 cups spring water
2 tablespoons butter
1 teaspoon olive oil
1 large onion, chopped
1 clove garlic, minced
2 cups celery, chopped
4 cups vegetable broth 4 bouillon cubes, 4 cups water
1/4 teaspoon dried tarragon
1/2 teaspoon dried sage
1 teaspoon dried thyme
1 dash cayenne pepper
1 dash nutmeg
1 dash sea salt

In a large soup pot, melt butter and heat oil. Add onion, garlic, celery, potatoes, and spices. Add water and bouillon to cover vegetables. Bring to a boil. Lower heat and simmer until vegetables are soft, for 20 minutes. Put into a blender or food processor for a creamy consistency. Serve hot.

COMPATIBLE with "A" and "Neutral" foods
*Optional for Working People: Same as Day One

DINNER:

Chicken Nuggets   4-6 servings

2 1/2 pounds boneless chicken breasts cut into 1-inch pieces
Olive oil for frying
1/2 cup cream (diluted with 1 cup spring water)
1/4 cup soy flour
1/4 cup grated Parmesan cheese
1 teaspoon paprika
1/2 teaspoon oregano

1. In a large frying pan, heat 1 inch of oil to 350°F.
2. Meanwhile, put cream in a bowl. In a paper bag, combine flour, Parmesan cheese, paprika, and oregano. Mix well. First dip chicken pieces in cream; then place about a dozen pieces of chicken at a time in bag and shake to coat.
3. Fry chicken in hot oil in batches, turning occasionally, for about 5 minutes, until crisp and golden brown. Drain on paper towels; serve hot.

COMPATIBLE with "B" and "Neutral" foods
OTHER DINNER OPTIONS: Same as Day One
DESSERT: "B" and "Neutral"

DAY TWENTY-EIGHT

BREAKFAST: Same as Day One

LUNCH:

Peking Chicken Salad*   4 servings

1 pound cooked (or fried) chicken; diced (or any kind of poultry)
2 seedless oranges, diced
2 tablespoons grated orange peel
2 cups mayonnaise
1 cup almonds, cut in halves
Dash cognac
Pinch nutmeg

    1. In a large bowl, combine all ingredients and mix well. Chill thoroughly. Serve on lettuce; garnish with orange slices.

COMPATIBLE with "B" and "Neutral" foods
*Optional for Working People: Same as Day One

DINNER:

Pizza Romana Blanca

A&B Pizza Dough and A&B Pizza Sauce (see basic recipe Day One or cookbook)
1 large onion, sliced
1 large green pepper, sliced
1/2 pound mushrooms, sliced
2 cloves garlic, grated
1/2 pound leek, chopped
1/2 pound sheep's milk cheese, such as Ricotta Salada or goat's cheese
1 cup sour cream
1 tablespoon fresh basil, chopped (or 1 teaspoon dried)
Dried oregano to taste
1/2 pound olives (any kind)
3 cups mozzarella, shredded

1. Prepare pizza dough and pizza sauce.
2. Preheat oven to 350°F.
3. In a small saucepan, cook onions in a small amount of olive oil until tender, but not brown. Add leek, 1 cup sheep's (or goat's) milk cheese, basil, and sour cream. Spread mixture evenly over dough.
4. Cut remaining sheep's milk cheese in cubes.
5. Top pizza with olives, pepper, onions, mushrooms, and sheep's milk cheese.
6. Sprinkle mozzarella and oregano over the pizza.
7. Bake on lowest shelf until crust is firm and golden brown at edges, 20–25 minutes. Cut into serving pieces and serve warm.

COMPATIBLE with "A" and "Neutral" foods
OTHER DINNER OPTIONS: Same as Day One
DESSERT: Same as Day One

Chapter 19

FOUR-WEEK EXAMPLE MENU
For People with Health Problems

LEVEL TWO

The A&B LEVEL TWO Chart was designed specifically for anyone currently experiencing health problems. LEVEL TWO was designed to help your BioChemical Machine build up its alkalinity on a daily basis. You have to make up for those years, probably decades, when you unknowingly decreased your *alkaline reserves*. Fortunately, this task is easier than you might initially think.

To make it easier to follow the LEVEL TWO CHART, we prepared a second color-coded version of the LEVEL ONE A&B Chart.

The color-coding clarifies which food items are base-builders *(yellow)*, healthy good proteins *(yellow and white)*, and healthy carbohydrates *(yellow and white)*.

The healthy acid-builders are *white;* the bad proteins are highlighted in *gray,* and the extremely-bad proteins are *red.* The unhealthy denatured ("new history") carbohydrates are also *gray.*

Discuss the A&B Method with your medical doctor. S/he will be happy to help you incorporate these principles into his/her prescribed treatment plan.

Don't be surprised to see the A&B Power Salad and optional Ramses Salad throughout this four-week example menu. They each emphasize a variety of leafy greens in addition to raw cauliflower, broccoli, spinach, and cabbage. These are vegetables most of us are used to eating cooked. Eaten raw, these are the types of food your Biochemical Machine is yearning for!

- Cauliflower is high in pantothenic acid and is called the "rejuvenation vitamin." It demolishes fat and plays a central role in the biochemical reactions within the body.

- Broccoli is rich in vitamin B_6, which converts energy reserves into sugar and gives immediate strength. Broccoli is gifted with the power to detoxify and to strengthen the immune system, as well as preventing cancer.

- White and red cabbage is rich in vitamin B_6.

- Spinach is rich in vitamin B_2, which regulates fat metabolism and sugar metabolism.

Your first culinary experience with this "power bowl" of food—seasoned with mayonnaise, vinegar, oil, salt, pepper, and herbs or other dressing and dips—will delight your taste buds and invigorate your body chemistry!

I offer the following twelve points as an overview to help you adopt the LEVEL TWO principles more easily:

(1) REMEMBER ESSENTIAL#1: Eat from group "A"—Eat from group "B" but as much as possible AVOID eating from both at the same meal as much as possible. Wait at least three hours before switching between "A" to "B" or vice versa. "Neutrals" may be eaten at any time with no waiting period.

(2) EAT SMART: The key to health and well-being is simple. 80% of your daily intake of foods should be base-builders (yellow), i.e., all kinds of (fresh) vegetables, salads, fruits, nuts, and healthy carbohydrates, such as potatoes, kale, bananas, dates, figs, honey and healthy olive or flaxseed oils (ideally, virgin oils).

(3) EAT HEALTHY: The other 20% should be base-building dairy products (yellow) or healthy acid-builders: "Neutral" dairy products (white), whole wheat products (white), brown rice

255

(white) or other "Neutral" foods—for example, legumes *(white,* correct preparation is vital!), "Neutral" meat *(white),* "Neutral" fish *(white),* or other foods that are *white* on the A&B Chart.

(4) THE KEY POINTS
- Vegetables, salads, and fruits should be eaten FRESH. Potatoes should be steamed in their skins.
- Variety is the spice of life!
- Make the "A&B Power Salad" or optional Ramses Salad the foundation of your daily menu. See the four-week example menus and cookbook. The best vegetables for increasing alkaline are the root vegetables—raw carrots, turnips, beets, and all sorts of top vegetables such as spinach, sprouts, beet tops, chard, celery, onion tops, watercress, broccoli, cauliflower, or any green vegetable that contains juice.

(5) START YOUR DAY RIGHT: Begin your day with whole milk and two apples each morning. Apples and milk are extremely detoxifying. They keep sugar levels steady and help ensure that your Biochemical Machine obtains sufficient fiber, vitamins, and minerals. And AVOID eating low-fat, fat-free, or skim milk products! They prevent your BioChemical Machine from obtaining vital vitamins and minerals.

(6) AVOID extremely-bad proteins *(red)*, such as cooked meat and bad proteins *(gray)*, such as cooked fish, and cheese below 50% fat, as well as ready-made foods and any foods with artificial additives ("B" column, *gray*).

(7) Try to replace extremely-bad proteins like cooked meat and cooked fish with "Neutral" meat and fish.

(8) Although it is recommended you omit cooked meat *(red)* and cooked fish *(gray)* completely; sometimes there's nothing as tasty as a juicy steak. Strive to balance such meals with fresh base-building "B" and "Neutral" fruits to compensate for the poisonous debris of the bad and extremely-bad proteins.

(9) LIMIT, if not ELIMINATE all white flour products such as white bread, noodles, spaghetti, pasta, and white sugar. They are unhealthy acid-builders. Replace them with whole wheat products such as wheat bread and wheat noodles, which are healthy acid-builders. YOU MAY EAT CHOCOLATE from time to time, also the A&B-Burger® but it must be eaten with compatible "A" and/or "Neutral" foods, never with "B" foods.

(10) AVOID low-fat and fat-free products. They contain sugars and chemicals that *wreaks havoc* with your BioChemical Machine.

(11) AVOID industrialized oil, margarine *(gray)*, and trans fat *(red)*. Replace them with healthy natural oils (olive oil, flaxseed oil) and butter *(yellow)*.

(12) AVOID alcoholic beverages like sweet wine, champagne, whiskey, rye, etc., BUT YOU MAY DRINK BEER (with "A" and/or "Neutral," never with "B") and, moderately, red wine.

REMEMBER THE BIG SEVEN ESSENTIALS

DAY ONE

1. BREAKFAST:

Milk & Apple
1–2 (better two!) medium-size apples (6 oz. = 250 g)
3–4 glasses of whole milk (1 glass 250 ml = 1/4 of daily requirement)

OPTIONAL: yogurt or buttermilk over diced apples

2. BREAKFAST:

It is recommended that people following LEVEL TWO eat two breakfasts each day to get back a healthy body and enhance recovery

Cottage Cheese with 2 Tomatoes
(Sliced with a of pinch sea salt; quantity to taste while following doctor's advice)

OPTIONAL: Cottage cheese or mozzarella with any kind of "B" fruits. "Neutral" cheese such as goat's milk cheese (feta) with olives; or anything else from the "Neutral" group that you would like.

LUNCH:

The A&B Power Salad, along with milk and apples, should be your number one food choice. The Power Salad is a must! The Power Salad can be eaten during the day with smoked salami (be careful that the salami is not precooked), smoked ham, or any other smoked, dried, or cured meat or fish.

259

From late afternoon on, you can eat the Power Salad with potatoes, (natural) rice, (wheat) pasta, or wheat bread with butter or mayonnaise. If you eat the Power Salad with wheat bread, potatoes, rice, or wheat pasta, you may also eat bananas, grapes, figs, and dates, as well as raisins, nuts, and honey ("A"), and, of course, anything "Neutral" at any time.

You can add any other vegetables you want. Remember: *variety is important!* There is no limit to vegetables, salads, sprouts, and herbs. You don't need to add ALL of the following suggested vegetables to your Power Salad, but it would be great if you did. By eating so many different vegetables and salads—your metabolism has it all!

A&B Power Salad

Lettuce (romaine, iceberg, limestone, red leaf, watercress, or any other lettuce, broken into bite-size pieces)
Tomatoes, sliced or diced into cubes
Carrot, chopped or sliced, quantity to taste
1/2 onion, chopped
1/2 to 1 cucumber, sliced or diced into cubes
Parsley, chopped, quantity to taste
Chive, or any other herb, to taste
Sprouts/soy sprouts to taste
1/2 green or red pepper, sliced or diced into cubes
Olives, quantity to taste
White and/or red cabbage, chopped, quantity to taste
Cauliflower, florets, quantity to taste
Broccoli, florets, quantity to taste
Spinach, chopped, quantity to taste

1. Cut up vegetables, small or large to taste. Combine all vegetables in a large bowl.
2. In a small bowl, combine olive oil, apple vinegar, and sea salt. Pour over salad.

> **TIP FOR WORKING PEOPLE:**
> *Locate a local deli where you can compose your Power Salads. If there is no salad bar around, eat apples and mozzarella or cottage cheese with fruits instead and save the Power Salad for dinner.*

> **HELPFUL TIP:** *Most people quickly tire of cutting up vegetables day in and day out. In order to have this vital food available at any time, prepare a huge air-tight bowl of raw vegetables sufficient for a couple of days. Vegetables don't perish quickly and can be kept refrigerated for several days. Chop or slice carrots and white and/or red cabbage and prepare cauliflower and broccoli according to your taste. Put chopped onions in a separate bowl that can be closed, so that your refrigerator will not smell like onions! Prepare (wash and cut) only a limited amount of fresh leafy greens/lettuce, since those perish very quickly. When you come home, you just need to take a bit from every bowl and mix it with oil, vinegar and sea salt.*

AFTERNOON SNACK:

2 Medium Apples sliced with any kind of cream cheese on slices.

OPTIONAL SNACKS:
Any other "B" or "Neutral" fruits with any kind of "Neutral" cheese
    OR
Goat's milk cheese (feta) crumbled with chopped olives on top of celery stalks.

261

LATER IN THE AFTERNOON:

Smoked Whiting with fresh lemon juice garnish

OPTIONAL:
Raw carrots, dipped in olive or flaxseed oil
    OR
Cauliflower dipped in olive-oil/vinegar/sea-salt dressing

OPTIONAL:
A&B Sandwich (whole wheat roll with mayonnaise, tomatoes, lettuce and onions)
    OR
1 slice whole wheat bread with 1/2 oz. butter,
1 medium tomato, sliced and 1 dash sea salt
    OR
1 slice rye-wheat or graham bread with any kind of cream cheese, and chives or other herbs and vegetables, chopped with a pinch sea salt
    OR
1 slice whole wheat bread with 1/2 oz. butter, and 1 1/2 oz. cured ham, or beef-salami (may not be precooked!) i.e., any other "Neutral" meat.

DINNER:

New Potatoes Marseilles*

5 small red-skinned (if possible, organic) potatoes, unpeeled
(Alternative: 1–2 New Jersey potatoes, russet potatoes, or any other type)
2–3 tablespoons butter, melted
1/4 cup fresh parsley, chopped   Sea salt to taste

1. In a vegetable steamer, bring water to a boil. Place washed potatoes over boiling water for 20 minutes until tender. Remove from heat. Place potatoes in a large bowl. Let stand until potatoes are cool enough to handle.
2. Cut unpeeled potatoes into 1/4-inch slices. Place on baking sheet, and sprinkle evenly with butter and seasoning and place as close as possible to the broiler until crusty and golden; approximately 10 minutes.

(Note: With Carbohydrates Chewing is Key!)

*Refer to the next page for An IMPORTANT note about diabetes and carbohydrates.

LATER IN THE EVENING:

1 Large Banana (chew!)

OPTIONAL:
Any other "A"- and/or "Neutral" fruits
And/or 1/4 oz. raisins
And/or almonds, brazil nuts *(yellow)*
And/or cashew, filberts, hazelnuts, walnuts, etc. *(white)*
And 3 tablespoons 100% natural honey

OPTIONAL:
Buttermilk or any "Neutral" cream cheese and "Neutral" milk product.

OPTIONAL:
Ricotta cheese with 3 tablespoons 100% natural honey (kills bacteria), and almonds on top.

DAY TWO

1. BREAKFAST: Same as Day One
2. BREAKFAST: Same as Day One
LUNCH: Same as Day One
AFTERNOON SNACK: Same as Day One
LATER IN THE AFTERNOON: Same as Day One

DINNER:

Ramses Salad with Whole Wheat Bread (or Wheat Pita Bread)

5–6 fresh hot peppers, such as jalapenos
2–3 large tomatoes
1 head of lettuce
6 large cloves of garlic
2 large onions
1 bunch cilantro
1 lemon, peeled
1 tablespoon coriander
1 tablespoon cumin
Sea salt to taste
1/2 cup apple vinegar
1/2 cup olive oil

1. In a food processor, combine all ingredients. Process until well blended to form a smooth pulp.
2. Serve Ramses Salad in small bowls; top with olive oil. Serve with whole wheat bread or wheat pita bread.

HELPFUL TIP: *In a jar, put remaining (leftover) Ramses Salad. Cover with olive oil, 2 inches above pulp (for conservation). Refrigerate for later use.*

LATER IN THE EVENING: Same as Day One

DAY THREE

1. BREAKFAST: Same as Day One
2. BREAKFAST: Same as Day One

LUNCH

Mozzarella with Tomatoes   2 servings

2 large tomatoes, sliced
1 ball of mozzarella, sliced
Fresh basil, quantity to taste
Lemon
Olive oil or virgin
Sea salt

1. Cut tomatoes and mozzarella in thin slices. Arrange on a plate.
2. In a small bowl, combine lemon and oil. Pour mixture over mozzarella and tomatoes. Add sea salt to taste. Garnish with fresh basil.

AFTERNOON SNACK: Same as Day One
LATER IN THE AFTERNOON: Same as Day One
DINNER:

Broccoli Milanese with Potatoes   4 servings

6-8 potatoes, unpeeled
4 stalks broccoli, washed and stems cut off
2 tablespoons butter
2 teaspoons fresh lemon
Sea salt to taste

1. In a vegetable steamer, place unpeeled potatoes over boiling water for 20 minutes or until tender. Keep warm.
2. Cut broccoli into individual florets. Place in vegetable steamer over boiling water until tender, covered.
3. In a small saucepan, melt butter. Pour this over hot broccoli. Season with sea salt. Serve with (peeled) potatoes.

LATER IN THE EVENING: Same as Day One

DAY FOUR

1. BREAKFAST: Same as Day One
2. BREAKFAST: Same as Day One
LUNCH: Same as Day One
AFTERNOON SNACK: Same as Day One
LATER IN THE AFTERNOON: Same as Day One

DINNER:

New Potatoes Marseilles   4 servings

5 small red-skinned potatoes, unpeeled
(Alternative: 1–2 New Jersey potatoes,
Russet potatoes, or any other type)
2–3 tablespoons butter, melted
1/4 cup fresh parsley, chopped
Sea salt to taste

1. In a vegetable steamer, bring water to a boil. Place washed potatoes over boiling water for 20 minutes or until tender. Remove from heat. Place potatoes in a large bowl. Let stand until potatoes are cool enough to handle.
2. Cut unpeeled potatoes into 1/4-inch slices. Place on baking sheet and sprinkle evenly with butter. Sprinkle with seasoning and place as close as possible to heat of broiler until crusty and golden, approximately 10 minutes.

COMPATIBLE with "A" and "Neutral" foods
OPTIONAL: 1–2 slices wheat bread with fresh butter, bacon and/or cheese above 60% fat (cream cheese, Camembert, Brie, cottage cheese, etc.), with raw vegetables and/or mixed salads
DESSERT Same as Day One

LATER IN THE EVENING: Same as Day One

266

DAY FIVE

1. BREAKFAST: Same as Day One
2. BREAKFAST: Same as Day One
LUNCH: Same as Day One
AFTERNOON SNACK: Same as Day One
LATER IN THE AFTERNOON: Same as Day One

DINNER:

Village Salad   2 servings

1 pkg. (8 oz.) feta cheese, cut into chunks
2 medium tomatoes, cut into chunks
1 large cucumber, cut into chunks
1 medium red onion, cut into chunks
1/2 cup A&B dressing (olive oil, apple vinegar, sea salt)

Toss all ingredients. Serve with wheat bread.

LATER IN THE EVENING: Same as Day One

DAY SIX

1. BREAKFAST: Same as Day One
2. BREAKFAST: Same as Day One
LUNCH: Same as Day One
AFTERNOON SNACK: Same as Day One
LATER IN THE AFTERNOON: Same as Day One

DINNER:

Cauliflower Soufflé Côte d'Azur   4 servings

1 large cauliflower, cored and cut into small florets
3 tablespoons olive oil
2 egg yolks
1/4 cup parsley, chopped
1 pinch sweet Hungarian (or regular) paprika
1 pinch nutmeg

1. Preheat oven to 350°F.
2. In a large saucepan, cook cauliflower in boiling salted water until just tender, about 10 minutes. Remove from heat.
3. Put cauliflower in a small soufflé oiled dish
4. Whisk two egg yolks with 2 tablespoons oil, nutmeg, and parsley.
5. Spread egg mixture over cauliflower. Bake until soufflé is golden brown, about 10 minutes.

COMPATIBLE with "A", "B", and "Neutral" foods

> *Note: Cauliflower (pantothenic acid) detoxifies cells and plays a vital role in the biochemical reactions within the body—and it enhances new skin growth and glow!*

LATER IN THE EVENING: Same as Day One

DAY SEVEN

1. BREAKFAST: Same as Day One
2. BREAKFAST: Same as Day One
LUNCH: Same as Day One
AFTERNOON SNACK: Same as Day One
LATER IN THE AFTERNOON: Same as Day One

DINNER:

Cabbage Budapest with Steamed Potatoes 4 servings

1 white cabbage, sliced
1 pound onions, diced
2 cups vegetable broth (or 2 cups water and 2 bouillon cubes)
2 cups heavy cream
1 cup sour cream
2 tablespoons butter
Sea salt to taste
2 teaspoon Hungarian (or regular) paprika
Soy sauce to taste
Potatoes, quantity to taste

1. For potatoes, see Day One.
2. In a large saucepan, sauté onions in butter until golden brown. Add vegetable broth or bouillon and sea salt.
3. Place cabbage in saucepan and cook for 15–20 minutes.
4. Remove from heat and drain cabbage.
5. Combine heavy cream and sour cream with paprika and season to taste. Sprinkle mixture over cabbage. Let stand 10 minutes.
6. Serve cabbage with (peeled) potatoes.

LATER IN THE EVENING: Same as Day One

DAY EIGHT

1. BREAKFAST: Same as Day One
2. BREAKFAST Same as Day One
LUNCH: Same as Day One
AFTERNOON SNACK: Same as Day One
LATER IN THE AFTERNOON: Same as Day One

DINNER:

DON'T FORGET TO LEAVE ADEQUATE TIME TO PREPARE ALL BEAN DINNERS. Soaking of the beans requires at least 3 to 4 hours and an additional 4 to 5 hours for cooking! Prepare the day before.

Ramses Beans and Ramses Salad

Old Egyptian recipe; beans should be eaten with Ramses Salad to ensure proper digestion. Optional: chopped onions, dressed with vinegar, sea salt, and cumin.

2 pounds small fava beans
1 pound skinless fava beans
1 pound Garbanzo beans (chickpeas)
1/2 pound yellow lentils
1 large bulb of garlic, crushed through a press
2 tablespoons dried coriander

1 tablespoon cumin
Sea salt to taste

1. Wash beans and lentils separately. In a big bowl, put fava beans, skinless fava beans, and Garbanzo beans. Cover beans with plenty of (distilled) cold water. Soak beans at least for 3 to 4 hours. Remove from water.
2. In a large saucepan, bring water to a boil. Add fava beans and Garbanzo beans. Cover with water, 4 inches above beans. Reduce heat. Check the water level, adding water if necessary. Simmer over medium-low heat for 4 to 5 hours, until soft.
3. Add lentils during last hour. Add garlic, cumin, coriander, and sea salt. Let stand for 30 minutes.
4. Prepare Ramses Salad from Day Two. Top Beans with Ramses Salad. VARIATION: Mash beans with mixer. Top with Ramses Salad.

LATER IN THE EVENING: Same as Day One

DAY NINE

1. BREAKFAST: Same as Day One
2. BREAKFAST: Same as Day One
LUNCH: Same as Day Three
AFTERNOON SNACK: Same as Day One
LATER IN THE AFTERNOON: Same as Day One

DINNER:

Eggplant Normandy   4-6 servings

2 large eggplants (or 4 small)
8 oz. mozzarella, sliced
6 cloves garlic, crushed through a press
4 small onions, peeled
2 medium tomatoes, pureed
2 cups olive oil
1 bunch parsley, chopped
1 bunch cilantro, chopped
Sea salt
Celery salt

1. Preheat oven to 300°F.
2. With a sharp knife, remove stem head of eggplants. Cut eggplants in 1/2 inch slices.
3. Chop cilantro and parsley. Puree tomatoes. Add garlic. Mix well.
4. In a large saucepan, heat olive oil. Place eggplants in oil. Fry until brown.
5. On a oiled baking sheet, place eggplant slices. Sprinkle them with tomato-cilantro-parsley mixture. Bake for 20 minutes, until crispy. Season to taste.
6. Put sliced mozzarella on top—heat to melt in oven.

LATER IN THE EVENING: Same as Day One

DAY TEN

1. BREAKFAST: Same as Day One
2. BREAKFAST: Same as Day One
LUNCH: Same as Day One
AFTERNOON SNACK: Same as Day On
LATER IN THE AFTERNOON: Same as Day One

DINNER:

Creamy Cauliflower Soup   4-6 servings

6 cups spring water with 6 vegetable bouillon cubes
2 medium cauliflower, cored and coarsely chopped
1 onion, chopped
1 clove garlic, crushed through a press
2 tablespoons butter
1 tablespoon olive oil
2 stalks celery, chopped
8 scallions, chopped
1/8 teaspoon nutmeg
1 teaspoon dried basil
1/2 teaspoon dried thyme
1 teaspoon dried marjoram
1/2 teaspoon celery or sea salt
1/8 teaspoon of fresh ground black pepper

In a large soup pot, melt butter and heat oil. Add scallions, onions, garlic, cauliflower, and celery. Season with sea salt to taste. Cook over medium heat for several minutes, stirring frequently. Add vegetable bouillon; bring to a boil. Add basil, thyme, marjoram. Simmer, covered, over medium heat until cauliflower is tender, for 10–15 minutes. Remove cover and cool slightly. In blender, process until soup is smooth and creamy. Add nutmeg to taste.

LATER IN THE EVENING: Same as Day One

DAY ELEVEN

1. BREAKFAST: Same as Day One
2. BREAKFAST: Same as Day One
LUNCH: Same as Day One
AFTERNOON SNACK: Same as Day One
LATER IN THE AFTERNOON: Same as Day One

DINNER:

Mushrooms Lyon   2 servings

1/2 pound mushrooms
2 tablespoons butter
1 tablespoon fresh lemon juice
Dash sea salt
Dash garlic powder
Soy sauce

1. Wash mushrooms; cut and discard ends from stems. Cut mushrooms into slices.
2. In a saucepan, melt butter. Add mushrooms, tossing lightly in butter, until soft. Add lemon juice. Season to taste.

LATER IN THE EVENING: Same as Day One

DAY TWELVE

1. BREAKFAST: Same as Day One
2. BREAKFAST: Same as Day One
LUNCH: Same as Day One
AFTERNOON SNACK: Same as Day One
LATER IN THE AFTERNOON: Same as Day One

DINNER:

Potato Salad d'Alsace   4 servings

6 new potatoes, unpeeled
Beef salami (may not be precooked!), diced into cubes
OPTIONAL: smoked fish, quantity to taste
1 fresh cucumber, sliced
1 large tomato, cut into small cubes
2 large pickles (sour or sweet dill), chopped into very thin slices
1/2 bunch chives, chopped
Scallions, to taste, chopped
1 onion, chopped
Mayonnaise and/or chunky Blue Cheese dressing to taste
Olive or any other natural oil to taste
Apple vinegar to taste
Sea salt to taste

1. In a vegetable steamer, place potatoes over boiling water for 20 to 30 minutes or until tender. Remove from heat. Place potatoes in a large bowl. Let stand until potatoes are cool enough to handle. Peel potatoes. Cut potatoes into 1/2-inch cubes.
2. Add olive oil, apple vinegar, vegetables, cucumber, (not precooked!) salami (or fish), and mayonnaise to potatoes. Mix well.

LATER IN THE EVENING: Same as Day One

DAY THIRTEEN

1. BREAKFAST: Same as Day One
2. BREAKFAST: Same as Day One
LUNCH: Same as Day One
AFTERNOON SNACK: Same as Day One
LATER IN THE AFTERNOON: Same as Day One
DINNER: Same as Day Five (Village Salad)
LATER IN THE EVENING: Same as Day One

DAY FOURTEEN

1. BREAKFAST: Same as Day One
2. BREAKFAST: Same as Day One
LUNCH: Same as Day One
AFTERNOON SNACK: Same as Day One
LATER IN THE AFTERNOON: Same as Day One

DINNER:

A&B White Pizza Four Seasons

2 cups whole wheat flour
1 tablespoon yeast
1/2 cup water
2 tablespoons olive oil
1 tablespoon butter

275

1 teaspoon sea salt
Broccoli, small pieces, quantity to taste
Cauliflower, quantity to taste
Mushrooms, sliced, quantity to taste
1/2 eggplant, sliced into 3/4 inch
1 large onion, sliced into rings
3 cloves garlic
Olives, quantity to taste
3 cups mozzarella, shredded
1 cup Ricotta cheese
1/2 cup heavy cream
1 teaspoon oregano, 1 teaspoon dried parsley, and 1 teaspoon basil

1. <u>A&B Pizza Sauce:</u> In a food processor, combine Ricotta cheese, garlic, cream, oregano, parsley, dried basil. Process until a paste forms. Slowly add olive oil; set aside.
2. <u>Pizza Dough:</u> In a medium mixing bowl, combine flour, yeast, olive oil, sea salt, and water. Stir mixture together; knead with your hands until dough is firm but moist. (If necessary, add more water, 1 tablespoon at a time.) Let dough rest for 1 hour.
3. Knead dough again with your hands. Cover and let rise for 20 minutes in a warm place.
4. Preheat oven to 350°F. Sprinkle whole wheat flour over greased baking sheet. Roll out dough and place on baking sheet. Spread pizza sauce evenly over dough. Top with broccoli, cauliflower, mushrooms, eggplant, onions, olives. Sprinkle mozzarella evenly over the pizza.
5. Place baking sheet on lowest shelf in oven (or the floor of a gas oven) and bake until crust is firm and nicely brown, 15–20 minutes. Serve warm.

LATER IN THE EVENING: Same as Day One

DAY FIFTEEN

1. BREAKFAST: Same as Day One
2. BREAKFAST: Same as Day One
LUNCH: Same as Day One
AFTERNOON SNACK: Same as Day One
LATER IN THE AFTERNOON: Same as Day One

DINNER:

Austrian Baked Potatoes "Arnold"   4 servings

4 large potatoes
Butter (1 tablespoon for each potato)
Sour cream
Parsley and chives
Sea salt
Aluminum wrap

1. With a sharp knife, make a lengthwise cut across each potato. Season potatoes with sea salt to taste. Top each potato with a tablespoon of butter. Wrap each potato in aluminum foil.
2. Preheat oven to 400°F. Place potatoes on baking sheet. Bake until tender, about 45 minutes to 1 hour.
3. In a bowl, mix sour cream with parsley and chives to taste. Serve hot.
4. Garnish with herbed sour cream.

LATER IN THE EVENING: Same as Day One

DAY SIXTEEN

1. BREAKFAST: Same as Day One
2. BREAKFAST: Same as Day One
LUNCH: Same as Day One
AFTERNOON SNACK: Same as Day One
LATER IN THE AFTERNOON: Same as Day One

DINNER:

Italian Stuffed Green Peppers   4-8 servings

1 cup natural (brown) rice
2 pounds mushrooms
2 middle-size onions, sliced
2 middle-size onions, cut in halves
8 green peppers (or 8 zucchini or 8 large tomatoes)
5 cloves garlic, crushed through a press (or garlic powder to taste)
1/2 bunch parsley, chopped
1/2 bunch cilantro, chopped
1/2 bunch dill, chopped
2 tablespoons butter or olive oil
1 large lemon, juice of
1 bouillon cube
1 pinch celery salt
1 pinch cumin
1 pinch saffron

1. In a small saucepan boil 2 cups water and add rice; reduce heat.
2. Cut mushrooms into small pieces.
3. Mix cooked rice, mushrooms, parsley, cilantro, garlic and dill.
4. In a large bowl, combine vegetable, rice mix and seasonings (except saffron and lemon). Blend well.
5. With a sharp knife, cut off tops of green peppers (or tomatoes or zucchini). Carefully, remove seeds and veins, leaving stems intact.

278

6. Stuff vegetable with mixture.
7. Preheat oven to 350°F. In a large baking dish, melt 2 tablespoons of butter (or oil), bake 2 onions, cut in halves, until softened. Arrange vegetables.
8. In a small frying pan, heat 1 cup of water and add 1 bouillon cube, saffron, and lemon juice. Add to vegetables. Bake until vegetables absorb most of the juice. Remove from oven. Add sour cream. Let stand, 20 minutes. Serve warm.

LATER IN THE EVENING: Same as Day One

DAY SEVENTEEN

1. BREAKFAST: Same as Day One
2. BREAKFAST: Same as Day One
LUNCH: Same as Day One
AFTERNOON SNACK: Same as Day One
LATER IN THE AFTERNOON: Same as Day One

DINNER:
Same as Day Eight (Ramses Beans and Ramses Salad)
(OPTIONAL: Ramses Salad with Wheat Bread)

LATER IN THE EVENING: Same as Day One

DAY EIGHTEEN

1. BREAKFAST: Same as Day One
2. BREAKFAST: Same as Day One
LUNCH: Same as Day One
AFTERNOON SNACK: Same as Day One
LATER IN THE AFTERNOON: Same as Day One

DINNER:

<u>Crispy Rice Balls St. Tropez</u>   4-6 servings

1 cup brown rice
1 1/2 tablespoons butter
1/4 cup olive oil
4 cups chicken broth (or 4 bouillon cubes,
dissolved in 4 cups water)
1/4 pound finely shredded mozzarella cheese
1/4 cup feta cheese
1 tablespoon parsley, minced
1/8 tablespoon freshly ground pepper
1/4 teaspoon grated nutmeg

3 egg yolks
Bread crumbs
Wheat or soy flour

1. Prepare rice (basic recipe). Let cool.
2. In a large bowl, beat 1 egg yolk. Add rice along with cheese, parsley, pepper, nutmeg. Blend well. Cover mixture and refrigerate at least 1 hour, until chilled.
3. In a small bowl, beat 2 egg yolks with 2 teaspoons water; set aside.
4. Scoop mixture. Shape rice with the palms of your hands into balls (1 1/2 inches). Roll balls in egg yolks. Coat balls with bread crumbs. Place rice balls around the mozzarella. Cover with plastic wrap. Refrigerate for 2 hours.
5. First roll rice balls in flour; then egg yolks; then breadcrumbs.
6. In a heavy frying pan heat 3 inches of oil to 375°F. Place chilled rice balls in hot oil. Fry, occasionally turning, for 3–5 minutes, until golden brown. Remove with a spoon. Drain on paper towels. Serve at once COMPATIBLE with "A" and "Neutral" foods

LATER IN THE EVENING: Same as Day One

DAY NINETEEN

1. BREAKFAST: Same as Day One
2. BREAKFAST: Same as Day One
LUNCH: Same as Day One
AFTERNOON SNACK: Same as Day One
LATER IN THE AFTERNOON: Same as Day One

DINNER:

Smoked Salmon and Feta Cheese   2 servings

3 ounces thinly sliced smoked salmon
1/4 teaspoon hot pepper sauce
Dash of lemon juice
8 ounces cream cheese, softened
1 cup fresh dill or parsley
3/4 cup grated feta cheese (about 3 ounces)

1. Preheat oven to 400°F. In a small bowl or food processor, combine cream cheese, feta cheese, lemon juice, and hot sauce. Blend well.
2. Cut smoked salmon into about 30 pieces. Spoon about 2 teaspoons of cheese mixture over pieces of salmon and top each with dill or parsley. Bake until cheese is softened, about 5 minutes. Serve warm.

LATER IN THE EVENING: Same as Day One

DAY TWENTY

1. BREAKFAST: Same as Day One
2. BREAKFAST: Same as Day One
LUNCH: Same as Day One
AFTERNOON SNACK: Same as Day One
LATER IN THE AFTERNOON: Same as Day One

DINNER:

Cauliflower Soufflé Côte d'Azur   4 servings

1 large cauliflower (cored and cut into small florets)
3 tablespoons olive oil
2 egg yolks
1/4 cup parsley, chopped
1 pinch sweet Hungarian (or regular) paprika
1 pinch nutmeg

1. Preheat oven to 350°F.
2. In a large saucepan, cook cauliflower in boiling salted water for 10 minutes. Remove from heat.
3. Place cauliflower in small soufflé dish greased with oil.
4. Whisk two egg yolks, with olive oil, nutmeg, and parsley in separate bowl.
5. Pour egg mixture over cauliflower. Bake until soufflé is golden brown, 20 minutes.

LATER IN THE EVENING: Same as Day One

DAY TWENTY-ONE

1. BREAKFAST: Same as Day One
2. BREAKFAST: Same as Day One
LUNCH: Same as Day One
AFTERNOON SNACK: Same as Day One
LATER IN THE AFTERNOON: Same as Day One

DINNER:

Potato Salzburg with Sour Cream   4-6 servings

10 medium-sized new potatoes
1/2 cup sour cream
1/2 bunch chives, minced

1. Preheat oven to 400°F.
2. Arrange potatoes on a baking sheet. Bake potatoes until tender. Place potatoes in a large bowl. Let stand until potatoes are cool enough to handle.
3. Halve potatoes.
4. Using a small spoon, scoop out a little bit of potato and fill cavity with 2 teaspoons sour cream.
5. Bake until heated through, about 10 minutes. Garnish with chives.

LATER IN THE EVENING: Same as Day One

DAY TWENTY-TWO

1. BREAKFAST: Same as Day One
2. BREAKFAST: Same as Day One
LUNCH: Same as Day One
AFTERNOON SNACK: Same as Day One
LATER IN THE AFTERNOON: Same as Day One

DINNER:

Oriental Lentil Soup   4 servings

1 1/2 cups lentils (already soaked for 3-4 hours)
2 cups vegetable or 2 chicken bouillon cubes in 2 cups water
8 cups (distilled) water
1 large onion, minced
1 clove garlic, crushed through a press
2 stalks celery, chopped
2 large carrots, chopped
2 tablespoons fresh parsley, chopped
1/2 teaspoon sea salt
1 teaspoon dried oregano
1 teaspoon sweet Hungarian (or regular) paprika
1/2 teaspoon dried thyme
3 tablespoons olive oil

1. In a saucepan, melt olive oil over medium-high heat. Add onions, tossing for 5 minutes, until crisp-tender.
2. Add garlic, carrots, and celery. Add seasonings and herbs; mix well, tossing for 3–4 minutes.
3. Add vegetable or chicken bouillon; cook for 3 minutes.
4. Add lentils and 8 cups hot water. Simmer over low heat for 60 minutes.

LATER IN THE EVENING: Same as Day One

DAY TWENTY-THREE

1. BREAKFAST: Same as Day One
2. BREAKFAST: Same as Day One
LUNCH: Same as Day One
AFTERNOON SNACK: Same as Day One
LATER IN THE AFTERNOON: Same as Day One

DINNER:

Broccoli Milanese   2 servings

4 stalks broccoli, washed and stems cut off
2 tablespoons butter
2 tablespoons fresh lemon juice
Seasoning with sea salt, to taste

1. Cut broccoli into individual florets. Place in vegetable steamer over boiling water until tender, covered, for 7 minutes.
2. In a small saucepan, melt butter and mix with lemon juice. Pour sauce over hot broccoli. Season to taste.

LATER IN THE EVENING: Same as Day One

DAY TWENTY-FOUR

1. BREAKFAST: Same as Day One
2. BREAKFAST: Same as Day One
LUNCH: Same as Day One
AFTERNOON SNACK: Same as Day One
LATER IN THE AFTERNOON: Same as Day One

DINNER:

Asparagus Salad   2–3 servings

1 head lettuce
1/2 head red leaf lettuce
1/2 pound fresh (or canned) asparagus
3 tablespoons olive oil
1 tablespoon apple vinegar or lemon juice
1 clove garlic, crushed through a press
1/2 tablespoon mustard
Sea salt to taste

1. Wash salad, dry, and break into pieces. Cut off and discard heavy ends from asparagus.
2. In a medium saucepan, cook asparagus in boiling salted water until tender, 3–5 minutes. Remove from water, drain well, and cut into 1 1/2-inch pieces. Combine with lettuce.
3. For dressing: combine oil, garlic, mustard, sea salt, and lemon juice (or vinegar) in cup. Mix well. Pour over salad.

LATER IN THE EVENING: Same as Day One

DAY TWENTY-FIVE

1. BREAKFAST: Same as Day One
2. BREAKFAST: Same as Day One
LUNCH: Same as Day One
AFTERNOON SNACK: Same as Day One
LATER IN THE AFTERNOON: Same as Day One

DINNER:
Same as Day Eight (Ramses Beans and Ramses Salad)

LATER IN THE EVENING: Same as Day One

DAY TWENTY-SIX

1. BREAKFAST: Same as Day One
2. BREAKFAST: Same as Day One
LUNCH: Same as Day One
AFTERNOON SNACK: Same as Day One
LATER IN THE AFTERNOON: Same as Day One

DINNER:

Artichokes Venetian   4 servings
4 artichokes
Several stalks celery
1 bay leaf
1 clove garlic, crushed through a press

1. Wash artichokes. Trim end of stems. Snip thorny tip off each leaf.
2. In a vegetable steamer, place artichokes, garlic, celery stalks, and bay leaf over boiling water; steam for 30–40 minutes. As soon as leaves can be easily removed, discard bay leaf, celery, and garlic. Serve with melted butter for dipping.

DINNER OPTION TWO:

Potato Soufflé   4 servings
4 large potatoes, steamed and 1/4-inch sliced
4 zucchini, 1/4-inch sliced
1 large onion, sliced
4 egg yolks
1/2 cup mozzarella, shredded
Herbs to taste
Fresh and/or dried parsley to taste
4 tablespoons butter or olive oil

1. In a vegetable steamer, place potatoes over boiling water almost until tender. Add zucchini. Cook until tender. Place potatoes in a large bowl. Let stand until potatoes are cool enough to handle. Peel and slice potatoes.
2. In a small bowl, whisk egg yolks. Mix well; set aside.
3. In a medium saucepan, cook onions in butter (or oil) until golden brown.
4. Put potatoes and zucchini in soufflé dish; sprinkle egg mixture over potatoes and vegetables.
5. Sprinkle shredded mozzarella on top. Bake for another 3 minutes. Reduce heat. Cover soufflé dish. Let stand 15 minutes. Sprinkle herbs over soufflé.

LATER IN THE EVENING: Same as Day One

DAY TWENTY-SEVEN

1. BREAKFAST: Same as Day One
2. BREAKFAST: Same as Day One
LUNCH: Same as Day One
AFTERNOON SNACK: Same as Day One
LATER IN THE AFTERNOON: Same as Day One

DINNER:

Classic Potato Soup   4 servings

8 peeled potatoes (medium to large), chopped into cubes
6–7 cups spring water
2 tablespoons butter
1 teaspoon olive oil
1 large onion, chopped
1 clove garlic, minced
2 cups celery, chopped
4 cups vegetable broth (optional: 4 bouillon cubes, 4 cups water)
1/4 teaspoon dried tarragon
1/2 teaspoon dried sage
1 teaspoon dried thyme
1 dash nutmeg
1 dash sea salt

In a large soup pot, melt butter and heat oil. Add onion, garlic, celery, potatoes, and spices. Add water and bouillon to cover vegetables. Bring to a boil. Lower heat and simmer until vegetables are soft, for 20 minutes. Put into blender or food processor for a creamy consistency. Serve hot.

LATER IN THE EVENING: Same as Day One

DAY TWENTY-EIGHT

1. BREAKFAST: Same as Day One
2. BREAKFAST: Same as Day One
LUNCH: Same as Day One
AFTERNOON SNACK: Same as Day One
LATER IN THE AFTERNOON: Same as Day One
DINNER:

Pizza Romana Blanca

Pizza Dough and Pizza Sauce (see basic recipe cookbook)
1 large onion, sliced
1 tablespoon olive oil
1 large green pepper, sliced
1/2 pound mushrooms, sliced
2 cloves garlic, grated
1/2 pound leeks, chopped
1/2 pound sheep's milk cheese
1 cup sour cream
1 tablespoon fresh basil, chopped (or 1 teaspoon dried)
Dried oregano to taste
1/2 pound olives (any kind)
3 cups mozzarella, shredded

1. Prepare Pizza Dough and A&B Pizza Sauce.
2. Preheat oven to 350°F.
3. In a small saucepan, sauté onions in olive oil until tender but not brown. Add leeks, 1 cup sheep's milk cheese, basil, and sour cream.
4. Spread mixture evenly over dough. Cut remaining sheep's milk cheese in cubes. Top pizza with olives, pepper, onions, mushrooms, and sheep's milk cheese. Sprinkle mozzarella and oregano over pizza. Bake on lowest shelf until crust is firm and nicely brown at edges, 20–25 minutes. Cut into serving pieces and serve warm.

LATER IN THE EVENING: Same as Day One

Chapter 20

QUICK SOLUTION:
THE A&B TEN-DAY EXAMPLE
Quick-Start Program for Healthy People

Holy Cow! Look what makes you thin. . . .Grapefruit doesn't really rev up your metabolism. Cabbage doesn't really light a fuse under stored calories. But milk will. This isn't a new food fad; this is science. Just ask Michael Zemel, chairman of the nutrition department at the University of Tennessee in Knoxville. He's found that milk turns down the tendency of your fat cells to store the day's calories, and increases the amount frittered away as heat. . . .
Readers Digest, July 2002, page 107 by Lisa Davis.

- Whole milk and apples along with the A&B Power Salad or the optional Ramses Salad is the foundation of the A&B 10-Day Quick Loss Program. For those who lack patience and want—for whatever reasons—to lose weight quickly, these foods make the process both healthy and easy!

- BETWEEN MEALS eat "Neutrals" such as nuts (but no "A"-peanuts) and seeds, cooked egg yolks (without the whites), and/or raw cauliflower, tomatoes or any vegetable dipped in mayonnaise, salad dressing, olive oil, apple vinegar, sea salt, pepper, cottage cheese, goat's cheese, or any other "Neutral" cheese along with any "Neutral" meat or fish.

- BE CAREFUL with "B" sausages! They are not pure meat but contain ingredients that will upset your chemistry. In excess, this will ultimately lead to weight gain.

- ELIMINATE any LOW-FAT or FAT-FREE products containing sugar and artificial additives. These chemicals interfere with your body's chemistry, the A&B principles and food chemistry.

- DRINK spring water or tea with cream. Avoid sodas, even those without sugar.

- IF YOU FIND YOURSELF GETTING HUNGRY during the day, eat milk and apples because a well-balanced blood sugar level curbs your appetite.

- Moderate jogging, workout or a brisk, or ½ to 1 hour "normal" walk (with emphasis on "each day") is mandatory.

DAY ONE

BREAKFAST:

Whole Milk & Apples
(Quantity to taste)

LUNCH:

Mozzarella with Tomatoes*   2 servings

2 large tomatoes, sliced
1 mozzarella, sliced
Fresh basil
Olive oil
Apple vinegar
Sea salt and pepper to taste

1. Cut tomatoes and mozzarella in slices. Arrange on a plate.
2. In a small bowl, combine vinegar and oil. Pour mixture over mozzarella and tomatoes. Add salt and pepper to taste. Garnish with fresh basil.

*OPTIONAL: *At work you may prefer to bring your food from home. Be sure to pack plenty of fruits from the "B" group—preferably apples—or any kind of salad similar to the A&B Power Salad. You can eat your salads and fruits with cottage cheese, goat or sheep's milk cheese, feta, mozzarella, cream cheese, Roquefort, ricotta, or anything from the "Neutral" group.*

IF YOU GET HUNGRY later during the day eat WHOLE MILK and APPLES because a well-balanced blood sugar level curbs your appetite!

293

DINNER:

There is no limit to the quantity of vegetables, salads, sprouts, and herbs you may eat. Your salads don't need ALL of the following ingredients just keep in mind, variety is important! Eating so many different vegetables and salads will keep your BioChemical Machine happy and healthy.

A&B Power Salad with Goat's Cheese *(or any other "Neutral" cheese)*

Lettuce (romaine, iceberg, limestone, red leaf, watercress, or any other lettuce, broken into bite-size pieces)
Tomatoes, sliced or diced into cubes
Cucumber, sliced or diced into cubes
Carrots, chopped or sliced
Cauliflower, chopped
Broccoli, chopped
White and/or red cabbage, chopped
Sprouts/soy sprouts
Spinach, chopped
Onions, sliced or diced into cubes
Scallions, sliced
Parsley, chopped
Chives, chopped
Oil to taste (olive, flaxseed, sesame, etc.)
Apple vinegar (opt: Balsamic) or fresh lemon juice to taste
Salt (sea salt, herb salt, Bio-salt) to taste
Pepper to taste

1. Cut vegetables. In a large bowl, combine all vegetables.
2. In a small bowl, combine oil, vinegar, salt, pepper, and chives.
3. Pour over salad.

Remember: For several servings put unused vegetables in air-tight container. Lettuce greens should be kept separately as they are more perishable. Dressing should be saved in a separate sealed container. Instant lunch and dinner!

DAY TWO

BREAKFAST: Same as Day One

LUNCH:

Broccoli Milanese*   2–3 servings

4 stalks broccoli, washed and stems cut off
2 tablespoons butter
2 teaspoons fresh lemon juice
Seasoning to taste

1. Cut each broccoli stem into individual florets. Place in vegetable steamer over boiling water until tender, covered, for 7 minutes.
2. In a small saucepan, melt butter; combine with lemon juice. Pour sauce over hot broccoli. Season to taste.

*Optional for Working People: Same as Day One

REMEMBER—IF YOU ARE GETTING HUNGRY...
Drink whole milk with apples.

DINNER:

A&B Power Salad (Same as Day One)

DAY THREE

BREAKFAST: Same as Day One

LUNCH:

Cauliflower Soufflé Côte d'Azur*   4 servings

1 large cauliflower, cored and broken into small florets
3 tablespoons oil
2 egg yolks
1/4 cup parsley, chopped
1 pinch sweet Hungarian (or regular) paprika
1 pinch nutmeg

1. Preheat oven to 350°F.
2. In a large saucepan, cook cauliflower in boiling salted water for 10 minutes. Remove from heat.
3. Put cauliflower in oiled soufflé dish.
4. Whisk two egg yolks, with 3 teaspoons oil, nutmeg, pepper, and parsley together in separate bowls.
5. Spread egg mixture over cauliflower. Bake until soufflé is golden brown, about 10 minutes.

*Optional for Working People: Same as Day One

Note: Cauliflower (which contains pantothenic acid) detoxifies cells and plays a vital role in the biochemical reactions within the body—and it enhances new skin production and glow..

REMEMBER—IF YOU ARE GETTING HUNGRY...
Drink whole milk with apples.

DINNER:

A&B Power Salad (Same as Day One)

DAY FOUR

BREAKFAST: Same as Day One

LUNCH:

Sylvia's Tuna Salad*   2 servings

1 (6 1/2 ounce) can tuna (in oil or water)
1/4 cup capers, either small size whole or large size halved
2 tablespoons onions, chopped
2 tablespoons mustard
1/2 cup pickled dill or sweet cucumber, diced
1/3 cup parsley, chopped
Olive oil, quantity to taste
1 teaspoon fresh lemon juice (or apple vinegar)
1/4 teaspoon pepper
Sea salt to taste
Garlic salt to taste

In a medium bowl, drain tuna then mash with oil and mustard. Add onions, lemon juice, pickled cucumber, ½ the capers, salt and pepper. Mix well. Serve on lettuce. Garnish with remaining capers or pickled cucumber slices.

*Optional for Working People: Same as Day One

DINNER:

A&B Power Salad (Same as Day One)

DAY FIVE

BREAKFAST: Same as Day One

LUNCH:

Roast Chicken Hawaii*   4 servings

1 whole chicken, about 3 pounds
2 tablespoons butter
2 tablespoons olive oil
1 cup pineapple, diced
1 teaspoon dried thyme
Sea salt and pepper to taste

1. Preheat oven to 350°F. Season chicken inside and out with salt and pepper. Place 1/2 teaspoon thyme in cavity. Tie legs together and rub butter over skin. Place in a large roasting pan with water.
2. Roast chicken for 15 minutes. Arrange diced pineapple around chicken. Sprinkle remaining thyme over chicken. Pour dry white wine over all and bake 1 hour and 15 minutes. Add water (or diluted cream) as soon as wine evaporates.

*Optional for Working People: Same as Day One or fried chicken.

REMEMBER—IF YOU ARE GETTING HUNGRY...
Drink whole milk with apples.

DINNER:

A&B Power Salad (Same as Day One)

DAY SIX

BREAKFAST: Same as Day One

LUNCH:

Mozzarella with Tomatoes*   2 servings

2 large tomatoes, sliced
1 pound mozzarella, sliced
Fresh basil
Apple vinegar to taste
Olive oil to taste
Sea salt to taste
Pepper to taste

1. Cut tomatoes and mozzarella in thin slices. Arrange on a plate.
2. In a small bowl, combine vinegar and oil. Pour mixture over mozzarella and tomatoes. Add salt and pepper to taste. Garnish with fresh basil.

*Optional for Working People: Same as Day One
REMEMBER—IF YOU ARE GETTING HUNGRY...
Drink whole milk with apples.

DINNER:

A&B Power Salad (Same as Day One)

DAY SEVEN

BREAKFAST: Same as Day One

LUNCH:

Meatballs*   4 servings

2 pounds ground meat
2 onions, chopped
2 onions, sliced
2 celery stalks
3–4 cloves garlic
1/2 bunch parsley
1 large can Italian peeled tomatoes
Olive oil
Soy flour (as needed—see below)
Soy sauce, sea salt, pepper to taste
Celery salt, oregano, basil to taste

1. In a food processor or blender, combine chopped onions, celery stalks, garlic, parsley, salt, pepper, celery salt, oregano, and basil. Process vegetables. Process until a puree forms.
2. Mix vegetable puree into chopped meat; mix very well; add soy flour until it is still moist, but can form a ball by rolling mixture into 1 1/2" balls in palms of hands.
3. In a frying pan, combine butter and sliced onions until lightly brown. Add salt, pepper, oregano, parsley, celery salt, and basil. Mix well. Add Italian peeled tomatoes; chop while cooking. Add meatballs and cook (low), turning, about 1 hour. Add soy sauce to taste.

*Optional for Working People: Same as Day One

REMEMBER—IF YOU ARE GETTING HUNGRY...
Drink whole milk with apples.

DINNER:
A&B Power Salad (Same as Day One)

DAY EIGHT

BREAKFAST: Same as Day On

LUNCH:

Mushrooms Lyon*   2 servings

1/2 pound mushrooms
2 tablespoons butter
1 tablespoon fresh lemon juice
Dash sea salt
Dash garlic powder
Soy sauce

1. Wash mushrooms; cut ends from stems. Cut mushrooms into slices.
2. In a saucepan, melt butter. Add mushrooms, tossing lightly in butter until soft. Add lemon juice. Season to taste.

*Optional for Working People: Same as Day One

REMEMBER—IF YOU ARE GETTING HUNGRY...
Drink whole milk with apples.

DINNER:

A&B Power Salad (Same as Day One)

DAY NINE

BREAKFAST: Same as Day One

LUNCH:

Mozzarella and Tomatoes*
(Same as Day One)

*Optional for Working People: Same as Day One

*REMEMBER—IF YOU ARE GETTING HUNGRY...
Drink whole milk with apples.*

DINNER:

Chef Salad

Lettuce (quantity to taste)
Tomatoes, sliced or diced into cubes
Cucumbers, thinly sliced
Broccoli, sliced
Cauliflower, sliced
Carrots, thinly sliced
Onions, sliced or diced into cubes
1–2 boiled whole eggs, sliced
Swiss cheese, thinly sliced
Smoked ham, sliced
Cooked turkey or chicken, rectangular slices
Olive oil to taste
Apple vinegar to taste
Salt to taste, Pepper to taste
Mayonnaise (OPTIONAL: dip or salad dressing)

Cut up vegetables. In a large bowl, combine all vegetables, smoked and/or cooked ham, cooked turkey, or chicken. Add oil, vinegar, salt, and pepper. Add mayonnaise, dip, or dressing. Save leftovers—without dressing for other lunches/dinners.

302

DAY TEN

BREAKFAST: Same as Day One

LUNCH:

Swiss Cheese Salad*   2–3 servings

1/2 pound Swiss cheese, thinly strips
2 medium onions, thinly sliced into rings
Olive oil to taste
Apple vinegar to taste
Salt to taste
Pepper to taste

In a medium bowl, combine all ingredients. Add salt and pepper to taste. Mix well.

*Optional for Working People: Same as Day One

REMEMBER—IF YOU ARE GETTING HUNGRY...
Drink whole milk with apples.

DINNER:

A&B Power Salad (Same as Day One)

Chapter 21

DIABETES:
It's Not About Food—It's About Cells!

Having Diabetes means your BioChemical Machine has been seriously damaged over the course of many years of (unknowingly) poisoning yourself. The BioChemical Machine is (or is almost) "out of order." Slowly but surely, one "spare part" (organs) after the other reduces its ability to function properly. Your BioChemical Machine makes little or no insulin and can not get blood sugar into the cells. As a result, the body doesn't receive the fuel it needs causing a high blood sugar count. This is one of the main reasons why diabetics are extremely tired and always desiring sleep. *In short, The BioChemical Machine needs repair! The type of repair can only be accomplished through the body's cells.*

However, the word "sugar" is misleading. Just as fat doesn't make fat, it is not the ordinary "sugar" that causes "sugar." Diabetes is the result of many years of abuse of your BioChemical Machine. That's why you have a very high blood sugar level after eating carbohydrates. The healthier you become the better your sugar level gets, because you are improving the ability of your BioChemical Machine to cope with carbohydrates. Therefore, in getting blood sugar into the cells again, your energy will be back and so will a fulfilling lifestyle.

At one point in time, my husband had a 570 blood sugar level (almost comatose) and his liver, kidney, heart and lungs were not working properly anymore. Basically, he was dying. However, it was his illness (and my fear of his impending death) that lead to cognitions that will revolutionize the treatment/cure of diabetes, and to my discovery that M.D.s are prescribing the wrong diet. They are keeping the sugar level artificially low by advising foods that are not supposed to raise the insulin level; such as bad proteins ("B" column) or even white bread (gray-colored in the "A" column).

Yet, keeping the blood-sugar level low does NOT heal a damaged BioChemical Machine. As behind "controlling the rise of the insulin level" the illness itself is progressing (if not raging) and the BioChemical Machine will continue to deteriorate— step by step...

About Diabetes

Diabetes is a disease that affects the way the body uses food. Normally, the body turns food into sugar for energy. Then, the blood carries this sugar to cells throughout the body. There, insulin, a hormone helps turn sugar from food into energy for the body to work. But, when you have diabetes something goes wrong. The body makes little or no insulin and can't get blood sugar into the cells. As a result, the body doesn't get the fuel it needs and blood sugar stays too high. <u>However, the word "sugar" is misleading.</u> Just as fat doesn't make fat, it is not the ordinary "sugar" that causes "sugar." Diabetes is the result of many years of abuse of your BioChemical Machine. That's why you have a very high blood sugar level after eating carbohydrates. The healthier you get, the better your sugar level gets— because you are improving the ability of your BioChemical Machine to cope with carbohydrates. At the beginning, diabetics should eat potatoes and/or pizza moderately.

The physician's method of "controlling the blood sugar level" precipitates senseless diets. For example, the glycemic index (a ridiculous "science"—comparable to Middle Age philosophies such as, "don't take a bath and don't open the window...somebody might die") based its diets on counting exactly that: the rise of the blood sugar level after eating. So, it raises the same question again (as I said in the Introduction): What *are* they counting—since ALL food rises the insulin level (if not, we are talking corpses).

It is true that diabetics have problems digesting carbohydrates—IN THE BEGINNING even when eating according to the BioChemical A&B Method. Yet diabetics NEED to eat carbohydrates (and healthy oils, and of course, many apples and oranges) not only for energy (as carbohydrates and healthy oils are the # 1 and #2 energy suppliers)—but also to heal the BioChemical Machine. If they don't eat healthy carbohydrates (as they are usually told by their physicians), along with good proteins, their health will deteriorate to the point that they become tired to the extent that they would have only one desire: to sleep.

YET, with the BioChemical A&B Method you will be able to observe the step-by-step-healing process of your BioChemical Machine. Since diabetes is a disease that affects the way the body uses food, it goes hand in hand...the more the BioChemical Machine is healed, the better the body can make proper use of the foods ingested, especially carbohydrates—that turns it into sugar for energy. A steady blood sugar level means: your machine and its organs is starting to function correctly—and is healing!

Also, the BioChemical A&B Method enhances the effectiveness of medicine/insulin.

THESE ARE THE 14 MAJOR POINTS AS AN OVERVIEW:

- Stick to the BioChemical A&B Method religiously until your blood sugar level has become stable. Before breakfast it should not be higher than 140 (best around 100); after eating not higher than 220/230.

- Stick to the BIG SEVEN ESSENTIALS religiously.

- Incorporate the 12 major points from LEVEL TWO for people with health problems; see Chapter 19.

- Use the BioChemical A&B Charts LEVEL TWO. The color-coding clarifies which food items are base-builders (yellow), healthy good proteins (yellow and white), and healthy carbohydrates (yellow and white). The bad proteins are highlighted in gray, and the extremely-bad proteins are red. The unhealthy denatured ("new history") carbohydrates are also gray.

- You MUST walk (or work out) every day, because your "spare parts" of your BioChemical Machine need to get rid of the inner fat. Moderate jogging, a brisk or ½ to 1 hour "normal" walk is fine. It encourages blood circulation and supports the healing process of your BioChemical Machine.

- You MUST start your day with whole milk and/or yogurt and 2 apples (any brand is fine, Golden Delicious, Gala, etc.—they are all great). On the one hand this gets rid of the poison and helps your liver; and on the other hand it will keep your blood sugar level steady—while enabling your cells to heal your organs, starting with the liver, kidneys, vessels, etc. Plus, you will be getting all the fiber you need.

- Make sure that you do not get hungry over the course of a day! If you feel you are hungry…eat oranges (physicians will tell you not to eat them "because it rises the blood sugar level," YET they are healing the illness) and/or apples, or any other fruit, yogurt, mozzarella (with tomatoes, onions, apple vinegar and olive oil), or carrots dipped in olive oil, salads, or almonds. Eat small portions so that you are not burdening your body (machine) in the beginning, but eat 6 – 7 times or more a day.

- In the beginning and during the time that your machine is picking up its functions and healing the "spare parts"—try to eat your fresh vegetables raw, as well as anything else that can be eaten without cooking them.

- Don't eat carbohydrates before late afternoon because of the biological liver rhythm, see Chapter 5.

- Don't eat bad proteins (and definitely not extremely-bad proteins) when you first start the A&B Method. NOTHING that's gray or red on the BioChemical A&B Chart (no low-fat or fat-free items). Eat SMOKED fish, instead of cooked fish, as fresh smoked fish usually doesn't contain too many salt additives.

- Eat 80% "yellow" (as much fresh and uncooked as possible, except potatoes. (see high-grade protein, healing power and other "yellows" in Chapter 4), and 20% healthy acid-builders ("white" on the BioChemical A&B Charts), such as beans. (HOWEVER, you must follow the instructions in regard to cooking beans, see Chapter 16: Ramses Beans and Ramses Salad tastes great and are healthy, eaten the A&B way).

- You can eat as soon as you feel that your blood sugar level has reached the average and is stable as described in the first bulleted point. You can eat also bad proteins and extremely-bad proteins—from time to time. HOWEVER, you must always eat a bad protein, such as fried chicken or turkey accompanied by oranges and/or apples, or other "Neutral" and/or "B" fruits, and/or with the A&B Power Salad (or other fresh salads)—but NEVER with anything from the "A" group (including "A" fruit).

- Try not to eat bad proteins with cooked vegetables (tastes good, I know, but not much of what your cells need is left after heating.

- Always check the brands you buy. For example, there is fresh mozzarella with almost no salt, which is preferred. If you buy feta cheese put it in (warm and later cold) water to get rid of "bad salt." As soon as the salt is washed away, use new water and add SEA SALT (huge difference) according to your taste. Buy wheat bread made with yeast and sea salt (yes it's out there) and whole grain bread—NO white bread (even if it's "organic"!).

- Keep in mind; you will NEVER be able to go back to your "old eating habits," which are the main reason you became diabetic. If you *do* return to chemically wrong eating habits, it may take a while before you feel the illness coming back. In my husband's case, after he didn't need insulin any longer, he went back to his old eating habits and it took from October to April—then all of a sudden the blood sugar level was "jumping," and he got scared. Ever since then he's eating biochemically right and the damage reversal doesn't take as long to show improvement, only about 6-8 weeks.

THE FOLLOWING ARE THE "USUAL MEAL RULES" FOR DIABETICS:

- <u>BREAKFAST</u> Milk & Apple Therapy

- <u>IN BETWEEN SNACKS</u>: fruits, fresh vegetables, yogurt and almonds

- <u>LUNCH</u>: Mozzarella (fresh!) with organic tomatoes and a dressing of apple vinegar, olive oil, sea salt. Optional: Smoked fish with fresh lemon and the Mini A&B Power Salad.

- <u>LATE AFTERNOON SNACKS</u>: fruits, especially apples and oranges, fresh vegetables, yogurt, almonds.

- <u>DINNER</u>: during the first weeks the A&B Power Salad or the A&B Ramses Salad WITH one slice of wheat bread in the beginning in order not to "overload" your machine. Over time the machine will be able to "work" better and you can increase the wheat bread to two slices. After 4 weeks, add potatoes. CHEWING for bread, potatoes, oat, or any other carbohydrate food IS VITALLY IMPORTANT!

313

- <u>AFTER DINNER SNACKS</u>: If you are hungry you can eat apples and/or oranges, and/or almonds, and/or olives until you go to sleep. However, if the olives are too salty, put them in warm water, overnight, until the salt is gone, add cold water AND sea salt to taste.

The A&B Power Salad and optional Ramses Salad are vital for your healing process. As I said in Chapter 19, they each emphasize a variety of leafy greens in addition to raw cauliflower, broccoli, spinach, and cabbage. These are vegetables most of us are used to eating cooked. Eaten raw, these are the types of food which are vital for the healing process.

- Cauliflower is high in pantothenic acid and is called the "rejuvenation vitamin." It demolishes fat and plays a central role in the biochemical reactions within the body.
- Broccoli is rich in vitamin B_6, which converts energy reserves into sugar for immediate strength. Broccoli is gifted with the power to detoxify and to strengthen the immune system, as well as preventing cancer.
- White and red cabbage is rich in vitamin B_6.
- Spinach is rich in vitamin B_2, which regulates fat metabolism and sugar metabolism.

Your first culinary experience with this "power bowl" of food—seasoned with apple vinegar, olive oil, sea salt (NO pepper), and herbs (NO ready-made dressings and dips during the first weeks)—will delight your taste buds and invigorate your body chemistry.

DAY ONE

1. BREAKFAST:

<u>Milk & Apple</u>
1–2 (better two!) medium-size apples (6 oz = 250 g)
3–4 glasses of whole milk (1 glass 250 ml = 1/4 of daily requirement)

<u>OPTIONAL</u>: yogurt or buttermilk served over bite-sized apple chunks

2. BREAKFAST:

<u>Fruits</u>
Oranges

LUNCH

<u>Smoked Whiting with Lemon</u>

OR
<u>Cottage Cheese with 2 Tomatoes</u>
(Sliced with a of pinch sea salt; quantity to taste while following doctor's advice).

OR
Cottage cheese or mozzarella with any kind of "B" fruits or any other "Neutral" cheese, such as goat's milk cheese (feta) with olives, or anything else from the "Neutral" group.

OR
Fresh Mozzarella with Tomatoes, onions, apple vinegar, olive oil and sea salt (NO pepper).

AFTERNOON SNACK:

2 Medium Apples with any kind of cream cheese spread on apple slices.

OPTIONAL:
Any other "B" or "Neutral" fruits with any kind of "Neutral" cheese
OR
Goat's milk cheese (feta) with olives or any other "Neutral" milk product.

LATER IN THE AFTERNOON:

Raw carrots, dipped in olive or flaxseed oil
OR
Cauliflower dipped in olive-oil/vinegar/sea-salt dressing

DINNER

The A&B Power Salad, along with milk and apples, should be your NUMBER ONE food choice in order to heal your BioChemical Machine, which is evident through a more and more steady blood sugar level. **REMEMBER**: "A steady blood sugar level means: your Machine took up its functions and is working again!

The Power Salad is a must. The Power Salad can be eaten during the day with salami (be careful that the salami is not precooked), smoked ham, or any other smoked, dried, or cured meat or fish.

From late afternoon on—you can eat the Power Salad with wheat bread, i.e., any whole grain bread. (Make sure you chew correctly, see 7 Essentials). After a couple of weeks, when the blood sugar level is already steady, you can eat it with potatoes, (natural) rice, (wheat) pasta, or wheat bread with butter (no margarine!). If you eat the Power Salad with wheat bread, potatoes, natural ("brown") rice, or wheat pasta LATER, you may eat also bananas, grapes, figs, and dates, as well as raisins, and honey ("A"), and, of course, anything "Neutral," such as almonds, etc.; at any time.

You can add any other vegetables you want! Remember: variety is important! There is no limit to vegetables, salads, sprouts, and herbs. You don't need to add ALL of the following suggested vegetables to your Power Salad, but it would be great if you did. By eating so many different vegetables and salads; your metabolism has it all.

A&B Power Salad

Lettuce (romaine, iceberg, limestone, red leaf, watercress, or any other lettuce, broken into bite-size pieces)
Tomatoes, sliced or diced into cubes
Carrot, chopped or sliced, quantity to taste
1/2 onion, chopped
1/2 to 1 cucumber, sliced or diced into cubes
Parsley, chopped, quantity to taste
Chive, or any other herb, to taste
Sprouts/soy sprouts to taste
1/2 green or red pepper, sliced or diced into cubes
Olives, quantity to taste
White and/or red cabbage, chopped, quantity to taste
Cauliflower, florets, quantity to taste
Broccoli, florets, quantity to taste
Spinach, chopped, quantity to taste

1. Cut up vegetables, small or large to taste. In a large bowl, combine all vegetables.
2. In a small bowl, combine olive oil, apple vinegar, and sea salt. Pour over salad.

HELPFUL TIP: *Most people quickly tire of cutting up vegetables day in and day out. In order to have this vital food available at any time, prepare a huge bowl of raw vegetables sufficient for a couple of days. Vegetables don't perish quickly and can be kept refrigerated for several days. Chop or slice carrots and white and/or red cabbage and prepare cauliflower and broccoli according to your taste. Put chopped onions in a separate bowl that can be closed, so that your refrigerator will not smell like onions! Prepare (wash and cut) only a limited amount of fresh leafy greens/lettuce, since those perish very quickly. When you come home, you just need to take a bit from every bowl and mix it with oil, vinegar and sea salt.*

318

LATER IN THE EVENING:

Fruits
And/or: Almonds, brazil nuts *(yellow)*=best! (At the beginning)

And/or: Cashews, filberts, hazelnuts, walnuts, etc. *(white).* And 3 tablespoons 100% natural honey to use as a dip.

OPTIONAL:
Buttermilk, yogurt or any other "Neutral" cream cheese and "Neutral" milk product

OPTIONAL:
Ricotta cheese, 3 tablespoons 100% natural honey (kills bacteria), and almonds. Mix cheese and honey; top with nuts—a great snack or dessert!

DAY TWO

1. BREAKFAST: Same as Day One
2. BREAKFAST: Same as Day One
LUNCH: Same as Day One
AFTERNOON SNACK: Same as Day One
LATER IN THE AFTERNOON: Same as Day One

DINNER:

Ramses Salad with Whole Wheat Bread (or Wheat Pita Bread)

5–6 fresh hot peppers, such as jalapenos
2–3 large tomatoes
1 head of lettuce
6 large cloves of garlic
2 large onions
1 bunch cilantro
1 lemon, peeled
1 tablespoon coriander
1 tablespoon cumin
Sea salt to taste
1/2 cup apple vinegar
1/2 cup olive oil

3. In a food processor, combine all ingredients. Process until well blended to form a pulp.
4. Serve Ramses Salad in small bowls; top with olive oil. Serve with whole wheat bread or wheat pita bread.

HELPFUL TIP: *In a jar, put remaining (leftover) Ramses Salad. Cover with olive oil, 2 inches above pulp (for conservation). Refrigerate for later use.*

LATER IN THE EVENING: Same as Day One

DAY THREE

1. BREAKFAST: Same as Day One
2. BREAKFAST:

Mozzarella with Tomatoes   2 servings
2 large tomatoes, sliced
1 ball of mozzarella, sliced
Fresh basil, quantity to taste
Lemon
Olive oil or virgin, Sea salt

1. Cut tomatoes and mozzarella in thin slices. Arrange on a plate.
2. In a small bowl, combine lemon and oil. Pour mixture over
   mozzarella and tomatoes. Add sea salt to taste. Garnish with fresh
   basil.

LUNCH: Same as Day One
AFTERNOON SNACK: Same as Day One
LATER IN THE AFTERNOON: Same as Day One

DINNER:

Broccoli Milanese with Potatoes   4 servings
6-8 potatoes, unpeeled
4 stalks broccoli, washed and stems cut off
2 tablespoons butter
2 teaspoons fresh lemon, Sea salt to taste.

1. In a vegetable steamer, place unpeeled potatoes over boiling water for
   20 minutes or until tender. Keep warm.
2. Cut broccoli into individual florets. Place in vegetable steamer over
   boiling water until tender.
3. In a small saucepan, melt butter. Pour this over hot broccoli. Season
   with sea salt. Serve with (peeled) potatoes.

LATER IN THE EVENING: Same as Day One

PART VIII

A & B
Cook Book

This cookbook has been created not only with a view toward good health, but for all lifestyles. There are recipes for LEVEL ONE and LEVEL TWO health conditions. You should choose the dishes according to the level you are using.

Special recognition is awarded to
Sylvia Bennett
for her development of the following recipes aligned for chemical compatibility of the body's biochemistry.

You can also order the companion to The BioChemical Machine, the cookbook by Sylvia Bennett
"$5 DOLLAR MENUS FOR TWO"
Ask your local bookstore if they carry it or order direct from our Web site at www.bigapplevision.com

"A"
Recipes

"A" Breakfast

Milk & Apples

Although both, Milk & Apples do not belong to "A", your day should start with milk and apples.

The best breakfast is indeed milk (or yogurt) with apples, because it is, first of all, detoxifying, but also you will be not hungry for many hours to come. You will feel as if you have eaten a complete traditional breakfast. Apples are high in fiber; a medium apple contains 9–10 grams of fiber; a good portion of the 20–35 grams you need every day. One glass of milk (250 ml) contains 8 grams of fat, which is a fragment of the 60–80 grams of fat that are healthy for a moderately active person. But remember: apples and milk are "B" and should not be used in combination with an "A" breakfast.

However, if you cannot instantly change your eating habits, then you will find, in the following options some ideas for a healthy "traditional" breakfast.

Classic Cereal Breakfast

1. In a large bowl, add cereal (if possible, without sugar).
2. Add
   a) Natural whole milk yogurt,
   b) Cream (diluted with water), or
   c) Sour cream.
3. Combine the cereal to taste: with bananas, blueberries, raisins, dates, dried figs, honey, and/or all kinds of nuts (including peanuts, because they belong to "A").

BREAKFAST OPTION #2: Bagel with cream cheese

BREAKFAST OPTION #3: Wheat bread/rye (toast) with butter and honey or jam/jelly/marmalade. If you don't like it so sweet, then choose a wheat bread/rye bread (toast) with butter or mayonnaise and slices of tomatoes, onions (or cucumber), and salt; or fresh bread with butter, cottage cheese, and/or cream cheese, Camembert, goat's milk cheese, sheep's milk cheese, egg yolk (only), chives, and salt.

Classic Muesli

1 tablespoon cottage or ricotta cheese (not low or no fat varieties!)
1 banana
2 tablespoons nuts, grated
2 tablespoons raisins (or dates)
1 tablespoon wheat bran
1 tablespoon fresh flaxseed, crushed
3 tablespoons wheat germ*

In a medium bowl, combine cottage or ricotta cheese and banana. Mix well. Add remaining ingredients.

*Wheat germ: Much too ugly of a name for a great and good tasting product which is full of vitamins, (especially vitamin E); 3 tablespoons a day will do "miracles" for your health.

Fruit Muesli

Banana (and/or fresh or dried figs, dried apples,
    dried plums, dried dates, raisins)
2 tablespoons flaxseeds, crushed
2 tablespoons flaxseed oil
6 tablespoons buttermilk
1 tablespoon honey
Walnuts, grated or chopped
1 1/2 cups cottage or ricotta cheese
1 tablespoon honey

1. In a medium bowl, combine fruit with flaxseeds and 4 tablespoons buttermilk.
2. In medium bowl, combine cottage cheese (or ricotta) with 2 tablespoons buttermilk, honey, and flaxseed oil. Spread mixture over muesli; top with walnuts.

Fresh-Grain Muesli

1–3 figs (or dates)
1/2 cup raisins, soaked in water for 5 hours
1/2 cup grain, oat or wheat flakes
1 cup cream
1 banana, mashed (or 1 cup blueberries)

1. In a medium bowl with water, soak raisins for 5 hours.
2. Drain raisins and combine all ingredients.

Fresh Herb-Grain Breakfast

1 cup cottage cheese (or ricotta)
4 tablespoons wheat germ
2 tablespoons sunflower oil
4 tablespoons sour cream
1/4 cup chives
1/8 cup chervil
1 pinch of herb-salt (OPTIONAL: sea salt)

In a medium bowl, combine ingredients. Serve with wheat bread.

DO NOT buy low, no, or fat-free cheeses or dairy foods. See cheese; fat free/low fat products, Chapter 16.

"A"
Lunches and
Dinners

"A" Pizza

In the following you will find two BASIC RECIPES you need for every type of pizza:

A&B PIZZA DOUGH and A&B PIZZA SAUCE.

1. A&B Pizza Sauce replaces the common but chemically incompatible tomato sauce.
2. A&B Pizza Dough should be made from whole wheat flour or frozen wheat bread dough (thawed as package directs).

A&B PIZZA DOUGH

Basic Recipe

2 cups whole wheat flour
1 tablespoon yeast
1 1/2 cups water
2 tablespoons olive oil
1 tablespoon butter
1 teaspoon sea salt

1. In a medium mixing bowl combine flour, yeast, oil, salt, and water. Stir mixture together with your hands until dough is firm but moist (if necessary, add more water, 1 tablespoon at time). Let dough rest for 1 hour.
2. Knead dough again with your hands. Cover and let rise in a warm place (20 minutes).
3. Preheat oven to 350°F. Sprinkle whole wheat flour over greased baking sheet.
4. Using a rolling pin, roll out dough on baking sheet. Arrange toppings.

A&B PIZZA SAUCE

Basic Recipe

1 cup ricotta cheese
3 cloves garlic
1/2 cup heavy cream
1 teaspoon oregano
1 teaspoon dried parsley
1 teaspoon basil
1 tablespoon olive oil

In a food processor, combine cheese, garlic, cream, oregano, parsley, and basil. Process until a paste forms. Slowly add oil; set aside until A&B Pizza Dough is ready.

Pizza Romana Blanca

A&B Pizza Dough and A&B Pizza Sauce (basic recipe)
1 large onion, sliced
1 large green pepper, sliced
1/2 pound mushrooms, sliced
2 cloves garlic, grated
1/2 pound leeks, chopped
1/2 pound sheep's milk cheese (or feta or goat's cheese)
1 cup sour cream
1 tablespoon fresh basil, chopped (or 1 teaspoon dried)
Dried oregano to taste
1/2 pound olives
3 cups mozzarella, shredded

1. Prepare Pizza Dough.
2. Prepare Pizza Sauce.
3. In a small saucepan, steam onions until tender but not brown. Add chopped leeks, 1 cup sheep's milk cheese, basil, and sour cream.
4. Spread mixture evenly over dough. Cut remaining sheep's milk cheese in quarters. Top pizza with olives, pepper, onions, mushrooms, and sheep's milk cheese. Sprinkle mozzarella and oregano evenly over the pizza. Bake at 350°F on lowest shelf (or the floor of a gas oven) until crust is firm and nicely brown at edges, 20–25 minutes. Cut into serving pieces and serve warm.

Mozzarella Pizza

A&B Pizza Dough and A&B Pizza Sauce (basic recipe)
3 cups mozzarella cheese (about 12 ounces), shredded
2 tablespoons pine nuts

1. Prepare Pizza Dough.
2. Prepare Pizza Sauce.
3. Spread Pizza Sauce evenly over dough. Top with mozzarella and pine nuts. Place baking sheet on lowest shelf in oven (or the floor of a gas oven). Bake at 350°F until crust is firm and nicely brown, 15 to 20 minutes. Serve warm.

Pizza Via Veneto

A&B Pizza Dough and A&B Pizza Sauce (basic recipe)
1 jar/can artichoke hearts
2 medium onions, sliced
1/4 cup vegetable or olive oil
3 cups mozzarella, shredded
1 tablespoon oregano, chopped fresh (or 1 teaspoon dried)
2 tablespoons olive oil

1. Prepare Pizza Dough.
2. Prepare Pizza Sauce.
3. In a large frying pan, cook onions in oil, stirring occasionally, until tender. Add artichokes, cheese, and oregano; set aside.
4. Spread Pizza Sauce evenly over dough. Top with artichoke hearts, mozzarella, and oregano. Drizzle remaining oil over pizza and bake at 350°F on lowest shelf (or the floor of a gas oven) until crust is firm and nicely brown at edges, 15–20 minutes. Serve warm.

Pizza Athena

A&B Pizza Dough and A&B Pizza Sauce (basic recipe)
1 1/2 cups feta cheese, shredded
Olives (any kind, quantity to taste)
3 cups mozzarella, shredded

1. Prepare Pizza Dough.
2. Prepare Pizza Sauce.
3. Spread Pizza Sauce evenly over dough. Top with feta and olives. Sprinkle mozzarella evenly over the pizza. Place baking sheet on lowest shelf in oven and bake until crust is firm and nicely brown, 15–20 minutes. Serve warm.

Pizza Venetian

A&B Pizza Dough and A&B Pizza Sauce (basic recipe)
1 large eggplant
2 cups mozzarella, shredded
4 cloves garlic, chopped or crushed
1 large onion, chopped (for eggplants)
1 large onion, sliced into rings
1 green pepper, sliced
1 teaspoon oregano
1 teaspoon basil
1 teaspoon parsley
1/2 cup olive oil

1. Cut eggplant into 3/4-inch quarters. Put eggplant in a strainer. Sprinkle sufficient salt over eggplant. Let stand until fluid is removed, 45 minutes. In a large saucepan, cook eggplant in hot oil until brown. Add onions and garlic, turning, until eggplant is nicely brown; set aside.
2. Prepare Pizza Dough.
3. Prepare Pizza Sauce.
4. Spread Pizza Sauce over dough. Top with pieces of eggplant. Sprinkle oregano, parsley, and basil. Top with mozzarella and onion rings. Place baking sheet on lowest shelf in oven (or the floor of a gas oven) and bake at 350°F until crust is firm and nicely brown, 15–20 minutes. Serve warm.

Pizza Milanese

A&B Pizza Dough and A&B Pizza Sauce (basic recipe)
1/2 pound mushrooms, sliced
2 large leeks, sliced
1 large onion, sliced into rings
1–2 peppers, sliced into rings
Olives (any kind, quantity to taste)
Sea salt

1. Prepare Pizza Dough and Pizza Sauce.
2. Spread sauce evenly over dough. Top with mushrooms, leeks, onion rings, pepper rings, and olives. Place baking sheet on lowest shelf in oven (or the floor of a gas oven) and bake at 350°F until crust is firm and nicely brown, 15–20 minutes. Serve warm.

A&B Four Seasons White Pizza

A&B Pizza Dough and A&B Pizza Sauce (basic recipe)
Broccoli, quantity to taste
Cauliflower, quantity to taste
Mushrooms, quantity to taste
1/2 eggplant, sliced and salted
1 large onion, sliced into rings
Olives (quantity to taste)
3 cups mozzarella, shredded

1. Cut eggplant into 3/4-inch quarters. Put salted eggplant on paper towels to drain liquid. About 45 minutes. In a large saucepan, cook eggplant in hot oil until brown. Add onions and garlic, turning, until eggplant is nicely brown; set aside.
2. Prepare Pizza Dough.
3. Prepare Pizza Sauce.
4. Spread Pizza Sauce evenly over dough. Top with broccoli, cauliflower, mushrooms, eggplants, onions, olives. Sprinkle mozzarella evenly over the pizza. Place baking sheet on lowest shelf in oven (or the floor of a gas oven) and bake at 350°F until crust is firm and nicely brown, 15–20 minutes. Serve warm.

"A" Pasta

It would be in your best interest to buy pasta made from whole wheat flour. (However, you can eat white flour from time to time, especially in restaurants, if health reasons are not your main concern.) Pasta should be served with mixed salads and/or may be eaten with bananas, grapes, fresh figs, fresh dates, dried apples, dried plums, dried figs, dried dates, raisins, and all kind of nuts (including peanuts). Beer, whiskey, rye and gin are compatible.

THE A&B WHITE SAUCE IS A BASIC SAUCE
THAT CAN BE USED FOR EVERY PASTA DISH.

A&B WHITE SAUCE
Basic Recipe

6 tablespoons butter
4 tablespoons whole wheat flour
1 cup heavy cream (diluted with 2 cups water)
Pinch of sea salt and freshly ground pepper
Pinch of grated nutmeg, optional

In a saucepan, melt butter over low heat. Slowly add flour as butter melts; stir until smooth. Pour in cream, stirring constantly for 15 minutes or until smooth and velvety. Increase heat and stir until sauce comes to a boil. Immediately, low simmer for 10 minutes more, stirring occasionally. Add salt, pepper, and nutmeg to taste. Whisk again until the sauce is smooth.

Rigatoni with Broccoli and A&B White Sauce

4-6 servings

1 pound rigatoni or fusilli
1 bunch fresh broccoli, washed, cut into pieces with stems cut off
1/2 cup chopped olives, black and green
1/2 pound fatty bacon, chopped
3 cloves garlic, minced or pressed
1/4 cup dry white wine
7-oz. can chicken broth (or 1 cup bouillon)
2 tablespoons butter
1/2 cup fresh Italian parsley, chopped
1 tablespoon basil
1/2 cup olive oil
1 cup A&B White Sauce

1. Prepare A&B White Sauce; set aside.
2. In a frying pan, lightly brown oil, garlic, and bacon for 10 minutes. Add wine and let simmer over medium heat for 5 minutes. Add broken-up broccoli, salt, and pepper to taste; let cook for 10 minutes. Add chicken broth and 1 cup A&B White Sauce; simmer for 5 minutes. Add olives, basil, parsley, and butter; simmer another 3 minutes.
3. While sauce is simmering, cook pasta in boiling salted water until tender but firm. Remove from heat and drain. Place in warm bowl and mix with broccoli sauce. Serve immediately.

Rigatoni à la Gondola   4-6 servings

1 pound rigatoni
5 pieces dried mushrooms
1 cup heavy cream
1/2 cup feta cheese, crumbled
Fresh oregano to taste
Fresh basil to taste
3 cloves garlic, crushed through a press
1/4 cup olive oil
Olives, chopped (quantity to taste)

1. In a food processor, crush mushrooms; set aside.
2. In a frying pan, cook olive oil; add garlic, oregano, basil, and heavy cream (2 minutes.) Add feta cheese; set aside.
3. In a large saucepan, cook rigatoni in boiling salted water until tender but firm. Remove from heat and drain. Pour mixture over rigatoni. Mix well. Sprinkle crushed mushrooms together with chopped olives over rigatoni.

Spaghetti à la Toscana   4-6 servings

1/2 pound spaghetti
4 onions, chopped
2 large cloves garlic, crushed through a press
1 1/2 pounds mushrooms, sliced
2 tablespoons butter
1/2 pound grated or shredded fresh cheese (above 60% fat)
1 cup heavy cream
1 teaspoon fresh basil, chopped
1 pinch sea salt
1 pinch pepper
1 teaspoon basil
1 teaspoon oregano

1. In a medium saucepan, cook onions and mushrooms in butter until softened but not brown. Add garlic, salt, and pepper to taste. Add fresh cheese. Cook until melted. Add cream. Mix well; set aside.
2. In a large saucepan, cook pasta in boiling salted water until tender but firm. Remove from heat and drain. Sprinkle cheese mixture over spaghetti. Drizzle fresh basil and oregano to taste.

Fettucine Alfredo   4-6 servings

1 pound fettucine
8 tablespoons butter, softened
1/4 cup heavy cream
1 cup grated mozzarella cheese
Freshly ground pepper

1. Cook pasta in boiling salted water until tender but firm. Remove from heat and drain.
2. Place fettucine in a warm bowl or on a serving platter. Add butter, cream, and half the mozzarella cheese. Toss fettucine noodles gently until they are evently coated. Serve immediately, topped with pepper and remaining mozzarella cheese.

Spaghetti à la Bell Paese   4-6 servings

1 pound spaghetti
2 large tomatoes
1 bundle fresh basil
Parsley to taste
3 sticks celery
4 cloves garlic, crushed or chopped
2 fresh green onions
1/2 tablespoon fresh oregano
Olive oil
Sea salt to taste
Pepper to taste
Seasoning to taste

1. Cut all vegetables in very small pieces (don't cook). Add lemon and olive oil. Mix well.
2. In a large saucepan, cook spaghetti in boiling salted water until tender but firm. Remove from heat and drain. Spread mixture over spaghetti.

Pasta di Paesano   4-6 servings

1 pound elbow noodles
Feta cheese (quantity to taste)
1 cup heavy cream
4 cloves garlic, crushed through a press
Fresh mint (quantity to taste), chopped
Fresh spinach (quantity to taste), chopped
Olive oil

1. Combine (uncooked) spinach, mint, feta cheese, cream, olive oil, and garlic; set aside.
2. In a saucepan, cook noodles in boiling salted water until tender but firm. Remove from heat and drain. Add mixture to noodles. Mix well.

Spaghetti with Four Cheeses   4-6 servings

1 pound spaghetti
2 oz. feta cheese
2 oz. cream Gouda cheese
2 oz. Gorgonzola (Italian soft blue cheese)
2 oz. cottage cheese
1/4 cup butter
Sea salt to taste

1. Dice all cheese, except cottage cheese, into 1/4 inch cubes; place in a bowl; set aside.
2. Cook pasta in boiling salted water until tender but firm. Remove from heat and drain. Place spaghetti back into the same pot and add butter and diced cheese.
3. Simmer over medium heat, stirring well until cheese is melted. Remove from heat and place in warm bowl. Sprinkle with cottage cheese and serve immediately.

Pasta à la Chinoise

4-6 servings

1/2 pound spaghetti
4 carrots, sliced
1 1/2 pounds mushrooms, sliced
4 scallions, sliced
2 stalks celery, sliced
Onion, sliced into rings
2 large cloves garlic, crushed or chopped
Butter to taste (or olive oil)
Soy sauce to taste
Cayenne pepper to taste
Ginger to taste
Sea salt to taste
Pepper to taste

1. In a large saucepan or wok, cook onions until golden brown. Gradually add carrots, mushrooms, celery, scallions, garlic, soy sauce, cayenne pepper, ginger, salt and pepper in butter or olive oil until brown; set aside.
2. In a saucepan, cook pasta in boiling salted water until tender but firm. Remove from heat and drain.
3. Add spaghetti to mixture. Mix well.

White Macaroni and Cheese

4-6 servings

1 pound macaroni
3 cups mozzarella, shredded
4–5 cloves garlic, crushed or chopped
1 teaspoon oregano
1 teaspoon thyme

1. In a large saucepan, cook macaroni in boiling salted water until tender but firm. Remove from heat and drain.
2. Combine oregano, thyme, and garlic and sprinkle over macaroni. Sprinkle mozzarella evenly over the macaroni.
3. Preheat oven to 300°F. Place macaroni in a greased baking dish. Bake until macaroni is nicely brown and crisp, about 20 minutes.

Pasta Parisian   4-6 servings

1 pound rigatoni (or any type of pasta)
1 large eggplant
1 cup ricotta cheese (or cottage cheese)
1/2 cup heavy cream (diluted with a little water)
1/2 cup olive oil
2 large cloves garlic, crushed or chopped
2 carrots cut into thin strips
2 celery stalks, cut into thin strips
4 onions, chopped
Soy sauce to taste
1 teaspoon oregano
1 teaspoon basil
Cayenne pepper to taste

1. Cut eggplant into 3/4-inch cubes. Put eggplant in a strainer. Sprinkle sufficient salt over eggplant. Let stand until fluid is removed, 45 minutes.
2. In a saucepan, cook pasta in boiling salted water until tender but firm. Remove from heat and drain.
3. In a deep frying pan or wok, cook onions, and garlic in hot oil until brown. Add eggplant. Spice with soy sauce, oregano, basil, and cayenne pepper. Reduce heat; cook, stirring occasionally, at least 1/2 hour. Add ricotta (or cottage) cheese and 1/2 cup heavy cream. Add mixture to rigatoni. Mix well.

Angel's Hair (Capelli d'Angelo)   4-6 servings
with Mushrooms

1 pound capelli d'angelo
20 whole button mushrooms, cleaned
1/2 pound butter
Freshly ground pepper
4 tablespoons grated mozzarella

1. Cook pasta in boiling salted water for 1 minute until tender but firm.
2. Sauté mushrooms in butter for 10 minutes or until soft. Add pepper.
3. In a large, warm bowl, place half mushroom mixture; add drained capelli d'angelo and toss gently.
4. Sprinkle in mozzarella cheese and toss again. Serve warm with mushrooms and butter sauce spooned over.

Angel's Hair Soufflé (Capelli d'Angelo)   4 servings

1 pound capelli d'angelo
4 egg yolks, separated
1/2 cup grated mozzarella
1 cup A&B White Sauce

1. Prepare A&B White Sauce; set aside.
2. Cook pasta in boiling salted water for 1 minute or until tender but firm. Remove from heat and drain.
3. In a mixing bowl, combine egg yolks and mozzarella cheese. Mix until stiff.
4. Mix in capelli d'angelo and blend thoroughly.
5. Pour mixture into a buttered soufflé dish. Bake at 450°F, or until soufflé puffs up. Serve immediately with A&B White Sauce.

Pasta "Decamerone"   4-6 servings

1 pound rigatoni (or any other type of pasta)
1 1/2 pounds mushrooms, sliced
1 can green peas
2 tablespoons butter
2 cups heavy cream
1 cup cream cheese
4 onions, chopped
2 large cloves garlic, crushed or chopped

1. In a medium saucepan, cook onions and mushrooms in butter until softened but not brown. Add peas (without fluid), garlic, salt, and pepper to taste. Add heavy cream and cream cheese. Mix well; set aside.
2. In a large saucepan, cook pasta in boiling salted water until tender but firm. Remove from heat and drain. Sprinkle mixture over pasta. Mix well.

Rigatoni with Garlic   4-6 servings

1 pound rigatoni
5 tablespoons olive oil
2 cloves garlic, minced or pressed
Pinch of sea salt
Pinch of freshly ground pepper
3 sprigs rosemary

1. Cook pasta in boiling salted water until tender but firm.
2. While pasta is cooking, fry garlic, rosemary, salt, and pepper in oil until garlic is golden brown. Add 2 tablespoons of the water in which the rigatoni is cooking; stir. Remove rosemary from oil mixture.
3. When rigatoni is cooked, remove from heat and drain. Place in a warm bowl; mix with the flavored oil and serve immediately.

Trenette with Pesto   4-6 servings

1 pound trenette
4 garlic cloves, crushed
2 cups fresh basil leaves, crushed
Sea salt to taste
1 teaspoon olive oil
1 cup grated mozzarella cheese
1/2 cup pine nuts

1. Crush basil leaves with a mortar and pestle, gradually adding salt and garlic cloves. When all the garlic and basil is thoroughly crushed, start to add mozzarella cheese. Continue to grind until all the ingredients form a fairly thick consistency. Dilute with olive oil. Now the pesto sauce is ready. Set aside.
2. Cook pasta in boiling salted water until tender but firm. Remove from heat and drain. Place
3. trenette in a warm bowl and add pesto sauce; mix thoroughly until all noodles are evenly coated. Serve immediately.

"A" Variety

Mushroom Soufflé   4 servings

1 1/2 cups whole rye flour or 1/2 cup whole wheat flour
1/2 pound butter
1/2 cup water
1 pound mushrooms, sliced
1 small onion, chopped
1 egg yolk
1 cup heavy cream
Sea salt to taste
Pepper to taste

1. Preheat oven to 350°F.
2. In a medium mixing bowl, combine whole rye flour or whole wheat flour, butter, sea salt, and 1/2 cup water. Stir mixture together with your hands.
3. Brush soufflé pan with butter before placing 2/3 of the dough in soufflé pan. Reserve 1/3 of the dough; set aside.
4. In a small saucepan, fry chopped onions. Add mushrooms, egg yolks, heavy cream, and spices. Let cook 10 minutes.
5. Place mixture over dough in pan. Cover soufflé with remaining dough. Bake until brown and crispy.

"A" Potatoes

The potato is full of vitamin C, calcium, and phosphorus, but the richest concentration of minerals is directly under the skin. Therefore, cook potatoes in their jackets (unpeeled in the vegetable steamer), instead of peeling them before cooking.

Austrian Baked Potatoes "Arnold"   4 servings

4 large potatoes
Butter (1 tablespoon for each potato)
Sour cream, or ready-to-buy fresh creamy Italian garlic dip,
or fresh sour cream dip without preservatives
Herbs, parsley and chives
Sea salt
Pepper
Aluminum foil

1. With a sharp knife, make a 1-inch cut across each potato. Season potatoes with salt and pepper to taste. Top each potato with a tablespoon of butter. Wrap each potato in aluminum foil..
2. Preheat oven to 400°F. Place potatoes on baking sheet. Bake until tender about 45 minutes to 1 hour.
3. In a bowl, combine sour cream with parsley and chives to taste.
4. Serve hot in or out of aluminum foil topped with herbed sour cream.

Stove-Top Potato Casserole   4-6 servings

4 large unpeeled potatoes, steamed and 1/4-inch sliced
4 zucchinis, 1/4-inch sliced
1 large onion, sliced
4 egg yolks
1/2 cup mozzarella, shredded
Herbs to taste
Dried parsley to taste
4 tablespoons butter or oil

1. In a vegetable steamer, place potatoes over boiling water until almost tender. Add zucchini. Cook until tender. Place potatoes and zucchini in a large bowl. Let stand until they are cool enough to handle. Peel and slice potatoes.
2. In a small bowl, whisk egg yolks. Add mozzarella. Mix well; set aside.
3. In a large frying pan, cook onions in butter (or olive oil) until golden brown. Add potatoes and zucchini. Sprinkle egg mixture over vegetables. Cook for another 3 minutes. Reduce heat. Cover pan. Let stand 15 minutes. Sprinkle herbs over casserole.

Potato Salad Bavaria   4-6 servings

4 large or 6 small unpeeled potatoes, (any type)
1 onion, sliced
1/2 bunch parsley, chopped
Vinegar to taste
Olive oil to taste
Sea salt to taste
Pepper to taste

1. In a vegetable steamer, place potatoes over boiling water until almost tender. Remove from heat. Place potatoes in a large bowl. Let stand until potatoes are cool enough to handle. Peel potatoes.
2. Cut potatoes into 1/2-inch quarters. Add oil, vinegar, salt, and pepper to taste. Mix well.
3. Serve hot.

Potato Salad d'Alsace   4-6 servings

6 new potatoes, unpeeled
Beef salami or smoked fish, dice into cubes, quantity to taste
1 fresh cucumber, sliced
1 large tomato, diced into cubes
2 large pickles (sour or sweet dill), chopped into very thin slices
1/2 bunch chives, chopped
Scallions to taste, chopped
1 onion, chopped
Mayonnaise and/or chunky Blue Cheese dressing to taste
Olive or any other natural oil to taste
Vinegar to taste
Sea salt, pepper and celery salt to taste

1. In a vegetable steamer, place potatoes over boiling water and cook until tender. Remove from heat. Place potatoes in a large bowl. Let stand until potatoes are cool enough to handle. Peel potatoes. Cut potatoes into 1/2-inch cubes.
2. Add oil, vinegar, vegetables, pickled cucumbers, salami (or fish), and mayonnaise to potatoes. Mix well. Serve hot or cold.

Potato Salad Vienna   4-6 servings

4 large or 6 small potatoes, unpeeled
1 can peas
4 carrots, chopped
1/2 bundle parsley, chopped
Mayonnaise to taste
Oil to taste
Vinegar to taste
Sea salt to taste
Pepper to taste
Garlic powder to taste

1. In a vegetable steamer, place potatoes over boiling water and cook until tender. Remove from heat.
2. Place potatoes in a large bowl. Let stand until potatoes are cool enough to handle. Peel potatoes. Cut potatoes into 1/2-inch cubes.
3. Add oil, vinegar, carrots, parsley, peas (drained), mayonnaise, salt, pepper, and garlic powder to potatoes. Mix well. Serve hot or cold.

Hungarian Potato Salad
with Creamy Dressing

4-6 servings

6 new potatoes, unpeeled
2 tablespoons butter
1 cup red cabbage, shredded
1–2 tablespoons mayonnaise
1/4 cup olive oil
1 large garlic clove, crushed through a press
1/2 tablespoon sea salt
1/4 teaspoon Hungarian (or regular) paprika
1 tablespoon vinegar
1/2 teaspoon dried thyme
Fresh ground black pepper to taste

1. In a vegetable steamer, place potatoes over boiling water and cook until tender. Remove from heat.
2. Place potatoes in a large bowl. Let stand until potatoes are cool enough to handle. Peel potatoes. Cut potatoes into 1/2-inch cubes.
3. In a small saucepan, melt butter. Pour butter over potatoes; add sea salt and paprika and mix well. Add cabbage; set aside.
4. Combine oil, vinegar, salt, garlic, celery salt, herbs, and mayonnaise. Blend well until dressing forms a paste. Pour dressing over potato salad.

Austrian Potato "Pancake"   4 servings

2 medium baking potatoes
1/2 small onion, chopped
1 tablespoon whole wheat flour
1/4 teaspoon baking powder
1/2 cup olive oil
1/2 cup sour cream
2 egg yolks
1 tablespoon minced fresh marjoram (or 1 teaspoon dried)
1/4 teaspoon sea salt
1/8 teaspoon freshly ground pepper

1. In a food processor, grate potatoes.
2. Combine flour, baking powder, and onion. Mix well with potatoes.
3. Combine marjoram, egg yolks, salt, and pepper. Beat until well blended and blend into potato mixture.
4. In a large frying pan heat oil over medium heat. Drop small portions of potato mix into hot oil and flatten with back of a spoon. Cook, turning once, until golden brown on both sides, about 5 minutes. Drain on paper towels. Top each pancake with sour cream.

New Potatoes Marseilles   4-6 servings

5 medium-sized potatoes, unpeeled
2–3 tablespoons butter, melted
1/4 cup fresh parsley, chopped
sea salt
Pepper

1. In a vegetable steamer, place potatoes over boiling water and cook until tender.
2. Remove from heat. Place potatoes in a large bowl. Let stand until potatoes are cool enough to handle. Peel potatoes.
3. Cut potatoes into 1/4-inch slices.
4. Place on baking sheet and brush evenly with butter. Sprinkle with seasoning and put as closely as possible to heat of broiler until crusty and golden, for approximately 10 minutes. Sprinkle parsley over potatoes.

Potato Salzburg with Sour Cream   4-6 servings

10 medium-sized new potatoes, unpeeled
1/2 cup sour cream
1/2 bunch chives, minced

1. Preheat oven to 400°F.
2. Arrange potatoes on a baking sheet. Bake potatoes until tender. Place potatoes in a large bowl. Let stand until potatoes are cool enough to handle.
3. Halve potatoes.
4. Using a small spoon, scoop out a little bit of potato and top with 2 teaspoons sour cream.
5. Bake until heated through, about 10 minutes. Garnish with chives.

Sweet Potato Bites   4 servings

1 pound sweet potatoes (approximately 2-inch diameter)
2 tablespoons olive oil
1/3 cup sour cream

1. Preheat oven to 400°F.
2. Scrub potatoes and trim ends. Cut into 1/4-inch rounds.
3. Brush a baking dish with oil. Arrange sweet potato slices in a single layer; brush tops with remaining oil.
4. Bake 15 minutes or until slices are golden brown on the bottom. Turn slices over. Cook until both sides are nicely brown, 10 minutes.
5. Top with sour cream.

"A" Rice Meals

In the following section you will find the BASIC RECIPE for cooking rice. The A&B White Sauce can be used for almost every rice dish.

RICE   2-4 servings

1 cup natural (brown) rice
1 1/2 tablespoons butter
4 tablespoons olive oil
4 cups chicken broth (or 4 bouillon cubes, dissolved in 4 cups water)

In a medium saucepan, melt butter over medium-low heat. Add rice and cook, stirring, 2–3 minutes. Add 2 cups of broth (or bouillon). Cook rice until fluid is almost absorbed. Add 1 more cup broth. Cook until fluid is almost absorbed, 4–5 minutes. Gradually, add remaining broth. Cook, continuously stirring, until rice is tender but firm, about 20–25 minutes. Remove from heat. Let cool.

OPTIONAL:

1. Bring 4 cups water to boil. Add some sea salt and about 1 teaspoon olive oil or butter, if desired.
2. Add 1 cup rice; stir until thoroughly blended with water. Reduce heat. Cover. Simmer about 40 minutes. Turn off heat. Fluff rice with fork.

A&B WHITE SAUCE

6 tablespoons butter
4 tablespoons whole wheat flour
1 cup heavy cream (diluted with 2 cups water)
Pinch of sea salt and freshly ground pepper
Pinch of grated nutmeg, optional

In a saucepan, melt butter over low heat. Slowly pour in flour as butter melts; stir until smooth. Pour in cream, stirring constantly for 15 minutes or until smooth and velvety. Increase heat and stir until sauce comes to a boil. Immediately, lower heat and simmer for 10 minutes more, stirring occasionally. Add sea salt, pepper, and nutmeg to taste. Whisk again until the sauce is smooth.

Crispy Rice Balls St. Tropez 4 servings

1 cup brown rice
1 1/2 tablespoons butter
1/4 cup olive oil
4 cups chicken broth (or 4 bouillon cubes, dissolved in 4 cups water)
Wheat or soy flour
Bread crumbs
3 egg yolks
1/4 pound finely shredded mozzarella cheese
1/4 cup feta cheese
1 tablespoon parsley, minced
1/8 tablespoon freshly ground pepper
1/4 teaspoon grated nutmeg

1. Prepare rice (basic recipe). Let cool.
2. In a large bowl, beat 1 egg yolk. Add rice along with cheese, parsley, pepper, nutmeg. Blend well. Cover mixture and refrigerate at least 1 hour, until chilled.
3. In a small bowl, beat 2 egg yolks with 2 teaspoons water; set aside. Mix well.
4. Scoop mixture. Shape rice with the palms of your hands into balls (1 1/2 inches).
5. First roll rice balls in flour; then egg yolks; then bread crumbs. Cover with plastic wrap. Refrigerate for 2 hours.
6. In a heavy frying pan heat 3 inches of oil to 375°F. Place chilled rice balls in hot oil. Fry, occasionally turning, for 3–5 minutes, until golden brown. Remove with a spoon. Drain on paper towels. Serve at once.

Rice Piazza San Marco 4-6 servings

Rice (basic recipe)
A&B White Sauce (basic recipe)
1 cup raisins, soaked in water for 5 hours
1/2 cup almonds, chopped
Walnuts

1. Prepare rice; set aside.
2. Prepare A&B White Sauce.
3. Mix rice with white sauce. Add raisins and almonds. Mix well. Garnish with walnuts.

Mediterranean Rice with Broccoli   4-6 servings

Rice (basic recipe)
1 bunch fresh broccoli stems cut off
1/2 cup chopped olives, black and green
1/2 pound Canadian bacon, chopped
3 cloves garlic, minced or pressed
1/4 cup dry white wine
7-oz. can chicken broth (or bouillon)
1 cup A&B White Sauce
2 tablespoons butter
1/2 cup olive oil
1/2 cup fresh parsley, chopped
1 tablespoon basil

1. Prepare rice. Remove from heat. Keep warm.
2. Prepare A&B White Sauce while rice cooks.
3. In a large saucepan, lightly brown oil, garlic, and bacon for 10 minutes. Add wine and let simmer over medium heat for 5 minutes. Add chicken broth and A&B White Sauce; simmer for 5 minutes. Add olives, basil, parsley, and butter; simmer another 3 minutes.
4. Mix rice into mixture.

Gilbert's Rice Salad   4-6 servings

1 cup natural (brown) rice
4 cups lettuce (or any other greens), chopped
1 tomato, quartered
1 medium onion, quartered
1/2 cup green olives, sliced
1/2 cup walnuts, chopped
1 tablespoon olive oil
Vinegar to taste
1 teaspoon dried basil
1 teaspoon dried oregano
Sea salt to taste
Cayenne pepper to taste
Pepper to taste

1. Prepare rice (basic recipe). Let stand until rice is cool enough to be refrigerated. Refrigerate 1 hour.
2. Add lettuce, onion, tomato, olives, oil, vinegar, walnuts, basil, oregano to cooled rice. Season to taste. Mix well.

"A" Couscous

Couscous Tunisian   4 servings

2 cups couscous
3 medium potatoes, cut in quarters
2 cups pumpkin pulp or squash, cut in cubes
5 carrots, cut in halves
2 celery stalks, cut 3 to 4-inches long
1 green pepper
1 red pepper
2 cloves garlic
1 large onion,
1 bunch coriander, sliced
Dried coriander
Cumin
Saffron
Sea salt
Pepper
3 vegetable, beef, or chicken bouillon cubes (diluted with 3 cups of water)
Butter
Oil

1. In a large frying pan, cook onions in oil, stirring occasionally, until tender. Add pumpkin or squash. Add garlic, coriander, vegetables, salt, pepper, dried coriander, cumin, and saffron. Let cook; stir occasionally. Add 3 cups bouillon. Let cook, until tender; set aside.
2. In a vegetable steamer, place couscous over boiling water. Cook until tender. Remove from heat but keep warm.
3. In a big bowl, place couscous. Pour vegetables and sauce over couscous. Serve warm.

"A" Soups

Classic Potato Soup   4-6 servings

8 peeled potatoes (medium to large), chopped in cubes
6–7 cups spring water
2 tablespoons butter
1 teaspoon olive oil
1 large onion, chopped
1 clove garlic, minced
2 cups celery, chopped
4 cups vegetable broth or 4 bouillon cubes, 4 cups water)
1/4 teaspoon dried tarragon
1/2 teaspoon dried sage
1 teaspoon dried thyme
1 dash cayenne pepper
1 dash nutmeg
1 dash sea salt

In a large soup pot, melt butter and heat oil. Add onion, garlic, celery, potatoes, bouillon, and spices. Add water and bouillon to cover vegetables. Bring to a boil. Lower heat and simmer until vegetables are soft, for 20 minutes. Put into blender or food processor for a creamy consistency. Serve hot.

Corn Soup   4-6 servings

2 fresh ears of corn (or one 10-ounce package frozen whole
  kernel corn, thawed)
1/4 cup onion, chopped
1 clove garlic, minced
1 tablespoon butter
1 cup chicken broth (or bouillon cube and 1 cup water)
Bottled hot sauce to taste
1/2 cup heavy cream
1/2 cup sour cream
1/4 teaspoon sea salt
1/8 teaspoon pepper
Cilantro, chopped
Parsley, chopped

1. If using fresh corn, use a sharp knife to cut off just the kernel
    tips from the cob.
2. In a blender or food processor combine half of the corn, sour
    cream, and heavy cream. Cover and blend or process until
    smooth, stopping machine occasionally to scrape down sides.
    Set mixture aside.
3. In a medium saucepan, cook onion and garlic in butter until
    tender but not brown.
4. Stir in blender corn mixture, remaining corn, broth, sea salt,
    pepper, and hot pepper sauce. Bring to boiling. Reduce heat and
    simmer for 20–25 minutes. Gradually stir in cream. Heat
    through, but do not boil. Season to taste. Garnish with parsley
    and cilantro.

"A" Desserts

Banana Cream

2 pounds ripened bananas
2 cups heavy cream, whipped
1/2 teaspoon vanilla
1/4 cup almonds, minced
Honey to taste
Raisins to taste

In a processor, combine bananas, honey with whipped cream and 1/2 teaspoon vanilla. Process until mixture is firm. Garnish with raisins; sprinkle almonds over banana cream; refrigerate.

Fried Bananas

Slightly firm bananas, cut in halves
Butter to taste
Almonds, chopped
2 tablespoons honey

In a frying pan, cook butter until golden brown. Add bananas. Fry until golden brown. Remove pan from heat. Sprinkle nuts, almonds, and honey over banana. Serve immediately.

Banana Flambé

1 slightly firm banana, sliced
2 tablespoons honey
2 tablespoons butter
Cognac to taste
Walnuts, chopped
Almonds, chopped

In a frying pan, add butter. Let cook until melted. Place banana. Top with nuts and almonds. Fry until golden brown. Add cognac. Burn off alcohol. Serve flambé with nuts.

363

Dessert "Amadeus Mozart"

1 cup cottage cheese or ricotta cheese
1/2 cup soaked raisins for 5 hours
1/2 cup heavy cream, whipped
2 egg yolks*
1/8 cup hazelnuts

In a medium bowl, combine ingredients. Mix well. Refrigerate. Serve chilled.

There is some danger of salmonella from uncooked egg yolk.

"A" Ice Cream

Banana Ice Cream

2 cups heavy cream, whipped
1 pound ripened bananas
2 tablespoons honey
1/2 cup walnuts, crushed

1. In a processor, combine whipped cream with bananas. Sweeten to taste.
2. Put mixture into a plastic bowl. Cover and freeze for at least 1 to 1 1/2 hours. Serve with whipped cream and decorate with walnuts.

Vanilla Ice Cream–Frozen Custard

2 cups heavy cream, whipped
4 egg yolks *
2 tablespoons honey
1 teaspoon vanilla
Walnuts

1. In a processor. combine whipped cream with egg yolks, honey, and vanilla. Process until mixture is foaming.
2. Put mixture into a plastic bowl. Cover and freeze for at least 1 to 1 1/2 hours. Serve with whipped cream and decorate with walnuts.

*There is some danger of salmonella from uncooked egg yolks.

Nut Ice Cream

2 cups heavy cream, whipped
4 egg yolks *
2 tablespoons honey
2 cups hazelnuts, crushed

1. In a processor, combine whipped cream with egg yolks, honey, and hazelnuts. Process until mixture is foaming.
2. Put mixture into a plastic bowl. Cover and freeze for at least 1 to 1 1/2 hours. Serve with whipped cream and decorate with hazelnuts.

*There is some danger of salmonella from uncooked egg yolks.

"A" Baked Treats

Cheese Pie

½ cup whole wheat flour
½ cup unbleached flour
4 tablespoons butter
½ cup plus 1 tablespoon cream
1 tablespoon honey

PIE FILLING
2 egg yolks
1 cup water
1 cup heavy cream
4 tablespoons honey
1 pound cottage cheese or ricotta cheese
1 package vanilla pudding powder
1 cup raisins

1. Preheat oven to 350°F.
2. Sift flour in a large bowl. Cut the butter into the flour by using a pastry cutter or two knives until it is the consistency of course corn meal. Knead dough well.
3. Add the honey, egg yolk, cottage cheese and vanilla pudding powder. Mix all ingredients until they are blended. Do not over mix. Add the raisins.
4. On a floured clean surface, role out dough until it is large enough to cover a pie pan. Use your rolling pin to lift the dough. Roll the dough around the rolling pin and place over the pie pan. Fit it in the pie pan and remove excess dough (save for another use).
5. Mix all the ingredients until blended. Spoon filling into crust.
6. Bake 30 minutes until it is golden on top. Let cool. Place in refrigerator until it thickens.
7. Serve and enjoy.

Blueberry Tarts

Prepare dough as in cheese pie
1 pound blueberries

1. Preheat oven to 350°F.
2. Knead dough. Place dough on cutting board. Cut into squares. Spoon blueberries on dough. Fold over into triangle.
3. On a greased baking sheet, arrange tarts. Bake for 10 minutes.

Raisin Tarts

Same dough as cheese pie.
1/2 pound ricotta cheese
1 cup raisins, soaked in water for 5 hours

1. Preheat oven to 350°F.
2. Combine ricotta cheese with raisins. Mix well.
3. Knead dough. Place dough on cutting board. Cut into squares, spoon cheese mix on dough. Fold over into triangle.
4. On a greased baking sheet, arrange tarts. Bake for 10 minutes.

Nut Cookies

1/4 pound rolled oats
1/4 pound butter
4 tablespoons honey
1 egg yolk
1/2 teaspoon baking powder
1/2 pound crushed hazelnuts

1. Preheat oven to 350°F.
2. Combine ingredients. Mix dough well.
3. On a greased baking sheet, place little portions of dough, about 1 teaspoon each. Garnish cookies with hazelnuts.
4. Bake cookies for 10 minutes, not too dark.

Banana Cake

1 cup whole wheat flour
1 teaspoon yeast
2 bananas, mashed
1/4 pound butter
3 tablespoons honey
2 egg yolks
1/4 pound walnuts, chopped

1. Preheat oven to 350°F.
2. Whisk butter, honey, egg yolks until foaming. Add whole wheat flour, yeast, and mashed bananas.
3. Place mixture in a greased and floured bread pan or baking pan. Sprinkle with chopped walnuts after slightly firm.
4. Bake cake for 20–25 minutes. Turn oven off. Leave for 2 – 5 more minutes. Remove, cool and cut into pieces.

Honey Pancakes

1/4 cup oil
2 egg yolks
2 cups whole wheat flour
1/2 teaspoon baking soda
1 pinch salt
1 1/2–2 cups water
1/2 pound ricotta or cottage cheese
1/2 cup raisins
1 tablespoon honey

1. Beat the egg yolks and oil together.
2. Combine flour, soda, and salt. Add to eggs.
3. Add water until batter is of desired consistency. Make pancakes on a hot griddle or frying pan coated with a little oil.
4. For topping, combine cheese, honey and raisins. Serve over pancakes.

"A" Bread

Flat Bread
(Makes 10 flat breads)

1 pound whole wheat flour
2 teaspoons yeast
1 teaspoon sea salt
5–6 tablespoons sunflower oil
1-1/2 cup water (or sour milk)
Sesame seeds (or caraway, sunflower, or poppy seeds)

1. Preheat oven to 350°F.
2. Combine ingredients, except choice of seeds. Mix well. Let stand at least 10 minutes.
3. Shape into flattered circles—about 6" in diameter, and slightly press seeds into dough.
4. Arrange bread flats on a greased baking sheet.
5. Bake bread for 10–15 minutes.

"A" A & B-Sandwiches

Replace any bread with rye, whole grain, whole wheat, potato, or Canadian oat bread.

A&B Sandwich

Whole wheat roll or 2 slices rye, potato bread, oat bread
Mayonnaise
Egg yolk, cooked, crumbled or chopped
Tomato, sliced
Lettuce, preferably dark or red lettuce, chopped

1. Spread mayonnaise on cut roll or bread slices.
2. Sprinkle egg yolk on mayonnaise
3. Add sliced tomatoes and sprinkle chopped lettuce evenly.

Pita L.T. and Onion

Pita bread
Mayonnaise
Tomatoes, sliced
Lettuce, chopped
Onions, sliced

1. Cut pita bread in half; spread mayonnaise.
2. Add tomatoes, lettuce, and onions.

Tramezzini "Romana"

2 slices whole wheat bread
Mayonnaise
Egg yolk, cooked
Lettuce, chopped
Tomatoes, sliced or chopped

1. Spread the bread with mayonnaise, sprinkle egg yolk, and add chopped lettuce and tomatoes.
2. Cut the bread diagonally.

A&B Fish Roll

1 whole wheat or rye roll
Marinated white herring
Sliced onions

Cut the roll; add herring and onions.

A&B "Oktoberfest" Sandwich

1 whole wheat roll
Smoked Salami
Mayonnaise or mustard
Pickles, sliced

Cut the roll. Spread the roll with mayonnaise or mustard. Add salami, and garnish with pickle slices (bread and butter chips).

French Roasted Bread with Garlic

1 baguette, whole wheat
Olive oil
Garlic, chopped

1. Preheat oven to 350°F.
2. Cut the baguette in half lengthwise
3. Pour oil over baguette and sprinkle the garlic evenly.
4. Toast the baguette in the oven.

B.L.T. Sandwich
(Either with Bacon, or Cured or Smoked Ham)

2 slices whole wheat bread
Lettuce, dark or red, quantity to taste
Tomato, sliced
Bacon

1. Spread the bread with mayonnaise.
2. Add lettuce, tomato, and bacon or ham.

Sandwich "Matador"

2 slices whole wheat bread
Mayonnaise
Sliced jalapeno pepper

Spread the bread slices with mayonnaise; add jalapeno pepper.

Bavarian Chives or Parsley Sandwich

2 slices whole wheat bread, rye, potato bread
Mayonnaise or butter
Chopped chives or parsley

Spread the bread with butter or mayonnaise; sprinkle chives or parsley evenly.

Smoked Salmon Sandwich

Smoked salmon, sliced
2 slices whole wheat bread or cut roll
Lettuce, dark or red, chopped
1 tomato, sliced
Dill, dried
Cream cheese

1. Spread the bread slices or cut roll with mayonnaise.
2. Add salmon slice(s).
3. Top with tomato slices and lettuce.
4. Top with cream cheese
5. Sprinkle dill evenly.

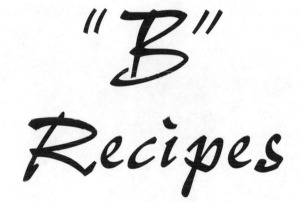

"B"
Recipes

"B" Breakfasts

1. Whole milk and apples. The best breakfast is indeed milk
    (or plain yogurt) with apples, because you will build a
    strong alkaline foundation for the day. (You can sweeten
    yogurt with sugar substitute.)

2. Scrambled (whole) eggs with bacon *(but without bread)*,
    and orange juice.

3. Scrambled egg yolks with bacon, *in this case, with bread*
    without orange juice.

4. Ham and eggs (without bread), and orange juice.

"B"
Lunches
and
Dinners

The following dishes can be served with any kind of vegetables; (except potatoes and kale); salads; and honey melon. Any kind of 'B" fruits; avocados with shrimp, vinegar, oil, and dill; shrimp cocktail with mayonnaise; mixed A&B salad; tuna salad; Waldorf Astoria salad; chicken salad with pineapple and mayonnaise; cheese of any kind; fruit salad; apple dessert with whipped cream; and ice cream with whipped cream and other desserts. However, for health reasons *you should eat strong acid-building cooked meat and cooked fish only with base-builders (fruits, salads, vegetables).*

"B" Poultry

Poultry should not be coated with sugar, syrup, or sugar containing sauces. You may coat your chicken with soy flour mixed with egg yolk.

Classic Roast Chicken   4-6 servings

1 whole chicken
1 medium onion, quartered
1 medium onion, sliced
2 carrots, thickly sliced
2 zucchinis, sliced
2 tablespoons butter
2 tablespoons olive oil
1 tablespoon soy flour
1 cup chicken stock or water with chicken bouillon cube
1 tablespoon dried thyme
Sea salt to taste
Pepper to taste

1. Rinse and dry the chicken.
2. Preheat oven to 350°F. Season chicken liberally with salt and pepper inside and out. Put small quartered onions and thyme inside cavity and tie legs together. Rub butter all over chicken.
3. Put oil in a large oval gratin dish or shallow roasting pan. Scatter sliced onion, zucchini, and carrot around the dish. Place chicken on top.
4. Roast chicken in oven until it is golden brown; about 25 minutes per pound.
5. Remove to a serving platter and cover with foil to keep warm.
6. Remove all but 2 tablespoons fat from pan. Place over medium heat, add soy flour, and cook, stirring, until thickened. Season with salt and pepper to taste. Strain into a gravy boat and serve with chicken.

Roast Chicken with Vegetables   4-6 servings

1 whole chicken, about 3 pounds, washed and rinsed
4 carrots, peeled and cut into 1-inch pieces
4 small onions, peeled and quartered
2 tablespoons butter, softened
1 pinch sea salt and pepper
1 cup (dry) white wine
1 teaspoon rosemary, crushed

1. Preheat oven to 350°F. Season chicken inside and out with salt and pepper. Place 1/2 teaspoon rosemary in cavity. Tie legs together and rub butter over skin. Place in a large roasting pan.
2. Roast chicken for 15 minutes. Arrange vegetables around chicken. Baste with wine and sprinkle remaining rosemary over chicken and vegetable.
3. Bake 1 hour and 15 minutes with pan drippings. Add water as soon as wine evaporates.

Roast Chicken Hawaii   4-6 servings

1 whole chicken, about 3 pounds, wash and rinse
2 tablespoons butter
2 tablespoons olive oil
Pineapple, diced
1/2 teaspoon dried thyme
Sea salt and pepper to taste
Dry white wine

1. Preheat oven to 350°F. Season chicken inside and out with salt and pepper. Place 1/2 teaspoon thyme in cavity. Tie legs together and rub butter over skin. Place in a large roasting pan with water.
2. Roast chicken for 15 minutes. Arrange diced pineapple around chicken. Sprinkle remaining thyme over chicken. Pour dry white wine over all and bake 1 hour and 15 minutes. Add water when wine evaporates.

Roast Chicken with Lemon
4-6 servings

1 whole 2-4 lb. chicken
1 garlic clove, split in half
1 lemon, quartered
1 small onion, quartered
Sea salt and pepper to taste

1. Preheat oven to 350°F.
2. Rinse chicken inside and out; pat dry.
3. Season inside and out with salt and pepper. Rub garlic over the skin; then place inside cavity. Stuff lemon and onion inside cavity. Tie legs together. Place chicken, breast side up, in a roasting pan with water.
4. Bake 1 hour and 15 minutes, until juices run clear.

Chicken with Mushrooms
6-8 servings

1 5 lb. roasting chicken
1/4 pound mushrooms, sliced
3 tablespoons parsley, chopped
3 tablespoons cilantro, chopped
1 egg yolk, beaten
2 tablespoons chopped parsley
2 teaspoons grated lemon peel
1 tablespoon fresh lemon juice
1 garlic clove, crushed through a press
Sea salt and freshly ground pepper

1. Preheat oven to 350°F.
2. In a large frying pan, melt 4 tablespoons of the butter over medium heat. Add onion and cook until tender, about 5 minutes. Remove from heat.
3. Add egg, parsley, cilantro, lemon peel, and 3/4 cup water to pan. Mix well. Add mushrooms. Put back on stove and let simmer until cooked. Set aside.
4. In a small saucepan, melt remaining 3 tablespoons butter. Add garlic and lemon juice; set aside.
5. Place chicken in a large roasting pan. Tie legs together. Season skin with salt and pepper. Brush with garlic butter and lemon.
6. Roast 2 1/2 hours, basting occasionally, until chicken is tender.
7. Serve with mushroom mixture on the side.

Ricotta Chicken   4-6 servings

1 roasting chicken, about 5 pounds
1 cup ricotta cheese
1 cup grated mozzarella
5 tablespoons butter
1 large onion, chopped
2 cups grated zucchini
1 garlic clove, crushed through a press
1 egg, beaten
1 teaspoon sea salt
1/2 teaspoon freshly ground pepper
1 teaspoon dried basil
1/2 teaspoon dried oregano
1/2 teaspoon dried marjoram

1. Preheat oven to 350°F.
2. Remove backbone and flatten chicken and place in a large roasting pan, skin side up. Starting at the breast, gently pull skin away from meat—leaving attached, but loosened.
3. In a large frying pan, melt 3 tablespoons of the butter over medium heat. Add onion and cook until tender, about 3 minutes. Add zucchini and cook until soft, about 3 minutes longer; remove from heat.
4. Add ricotta cheese, mozzarella, marjoram, egg, salt, and pepper to zucchini mixture. Mix well.
5. Spoon stuffing under the skin working over breast, thigh, and leg areas, smoothing it evenly under skin.
6. In a small saucepan, melt remaining 2 tablespoons butter. Add garlic, basil, and oregano. Brush chicken with seasoned butter. Roast 1-1/2 hours until tender and juices run clear. Baste every 20 or 30 minutes.

Parmesan Chicken   4-6 servings

1 chicken, 3 lb., cut up
3 tablespoons butter or as much as needed
2 tablespoons soy flour
1 cup sweet cream (diluted with water)
1/2 cup grated Parmesan cheese
1/2 cup shredded Swiss cheese
Sea salt and pepper

1. Preheat oven to 350°F.
2. Season chicken with salt and pepper.
3. In a large frying pan, melt butter over medium heat. Add chicken and cook, turning, until brown, about 10 minutes.
4. Sprinkle 1/4 cup of the Parmesan cheese over bottom of a well greased medium baking dish. Arrange chicken in dish.
5. In same frying pan, whisk soy flour into pan drippings. Cook, stirring for 1 minute. Gradually add cream and cook, stirring constantly, until smooth and thick. Lower heat and stir in Swiss cheese until melted. Pour sauce over chicken.
6. Top chicken with remaining 1/4 cup Parmesan cheese. Bake for 45 minutes to 1 hour, until chicken is tender.

Chicken with Spinach   4 servings

2 cups chopped cooked chicken
3 tablespoons butter
3 tablespoons soy flour
1 3/4 cups cream (diluted with a little water)
1 pound spinach, chopped
1 cup grated Parmesan cheese
10 slices Swiss cheese
1/2 pound mushrooms, halved
1 teaspoon sea salt
1 teaspoon pepper
1/4 teaspoon nutmeg
2 tablespoons water
Paper towels

1. Preheat oven to 350°F.
2. Place spinach in a large saucepan with 2 tablespoons water. Cover and steam until tender, about 3 minutes. Drain well; press between paper towels to squeeze out excess water. Transfer to a greased medium baking dish.
3. In a large saucepan, melt butter over medium heat. Stir in flour and cook, without browning, for 1 minute. Gradually whisk in cream and soy flour. Add salt, pepper, and nutmeg. Cook, stirring constantly, until mixture thickens and comes to a boil. Reduce heat to low, add Swiss cheese, and stir until melted.
4. Remove sauce from heat. Place chicken and mushrooms over spinach. Cover with sauce.
5. Sprinkle Parmesan cheese over chicken. Bake for 20 minutes, until bubbly and lightly brown on top.

Chicken Thighs with Vegetables   4 servings

8 pieces chicken thighs
1/2 cup grated Parmesan cheese
2 tablespoons butter
4 tablespoons butter, melted
1 cup grated carrots
1 cup broccoli, chopped
1 onion, chopped
Sea salt to taste
Pepper to taste
Oregano to taste

1. Preheat oven to 350°F.
2. Place chicken on a greased baking sheet. Sprinkle the chicken with butter and Parmesan cheese. Bake until chicken is tender, for 45 minutes to 1 hour.
3. In a frying pan, melt butter over medium-high heat. Add carrots, broccoli, and onion. Cook, tossing often until broccoli is crisp-tender.
4. Put vegetable mixture around chicken. Serve.

Chicken Wings and Blue Cheese Dip   4 servings

24 whole chicken wings
2–4 cups olive oil
4 tablespoons butter
2–5 tablespoons hot pepper sauce
1 tablespoon distilled white vinegar
Celery sticks
Blue cheese dip
Sea salt and pepper

1. Rinse chicken and pat dry. Halve wings at main joint and discard pointed tip of each wing. Season chicken with salt and pepper to taste.
2. In a large, heavy saucepan, heat 2 inches of oil to 375°F on a deep-frying thermometer. Cook the wings, in batches without crowding, until crisp and golden, about 10 minutes. Drain well on paper towels.
3. In a small saucepan, melt butter over medium-low heat. Stir in hot sauce and vinegar. Mound wings on a serving plate and pour hot butter sauce over them. Serve at once, with celery sticks and blue cheese dip.

Chicken with Herbs   4-6 servings

1 chicken, 3 lb. cut up
2 tablespoons butter
2 tablespoons chopped onion
2 tablespoons chopped parsley
1/2 cup dry white wine
1/4 cup grated Parmesan cheese
1 teaspoon paprika
1/4 teaspoon dried marjoram
1/4 teaspoon dried tarragon
1/2 teaspoon poultry seasoning
1/2 teaspoon dried oregano

1. Preheat oven to 350°F.
2. In a small saucepan, melt butter over medium heat. Add onion and cook until tender, about 3 minutes. Stir in parsley, oregano, poultry seasoning, tarragon, marjoram, and wine. Boil 5 minutes, until sauce is reduced by one-third.
3. Arrange chicken in a medium baking dish. Brush herb sauce over chicken. Sprinkle with Parmesan cheese and paprika. Bake 45 minutes to 1 hour, until tender.

Baked Chicken in Wine   4-6 servings

1 3 lb. chicken, cut up
2 large garlic bulbs, separated into cloves
3 celery stalks, cut into 1-inch lengths
1/4 cup olive oil
1/2 cup dry white wine
2 tablespoons parsley, chopped
2 tablespoons fresh basil, chopped, or 1/4 teaspoon dried
1/4 tablespoon freshly ground pepper
1/4 teaspoon hot pepper, crushed
3 tablespoons fresh lemon juice and 1/2 teaspoon grated lemon rind
Sea salt to taste

1. Preheat oven to 375°F.
2. Arrange chicken pieces in a medium baking dish, skin side up. Sprinkle garlic cloves and celery over and around chicken.
3. Mix wine, oil, salt, pepper, basil, lemon juice, and hot pepper. Pour over chicken. Sprinkle skinned lemon rind on top.
4. Bake, covered, for 40 minutes. Uncover and bake 15 minutes, until chicken is tender.

Chicken Veneziana 6-8 servings

2 chickens (about 3 pounds each), quartered
6 tablespoons butter
1/2 cup grated white Cheddar cheese
1 can (28 ounces) Italian peeled tomatoes, drained and finely chopped
1 1/4 cups soy flour
2 cups heavy cream
2 tablespoons olive oil
3 large onions, sliced
1/4 pound boiled ham, cut into thick strips
1/2 teaspoon white pepper and 1/4 teaspoon black pepper
1 teaspoon dried basil

1. Preheat oven to 350°F.
2. In a saucepan, melt 4 tablespoons of the butter over medium heat. Whisk in 1/4 cup of the soy flour and cook, stirring, 2 minutes without browning. Gradually whisk in cream. Bring to a boil then lower heat, cook, stirring until thickened. Season with white pepper. Remove from heat and stir in Cheddar cheese. Set aside.
3. Place remaining 1 cup soy flour and black pepper in plastic bag. Add chicken quarters and shake to coat.
4. In a large frying pan, melt remaining 2 tablespoons butter in oil over medium heat. Brown chicken in pan in batches, about 4 minutes on each side; remove to a large roasting pan.
5. Add onions to frying pan and cook 3 minutes, until softened. Add ham, tomatoes, sauce and basil. Cook 5 minutes. Pour sauce over chicken and cover. Bake 1 hour.
6. Arrange chicken on a large heated platter. Coat lightly with sauce. Put remaining sauce in gravy boat and pass around.

Chopped Chicken Liver   4 servings

1 pound chicken livers
2 tablespoons butter
2 tablespoons olive oil
2 hard-cooked egg yolks
2 medium onions, chopped
1 teaspoon minced garlic
1 teaspoon lemon juice
1/2 teaspoon freshly ground pepper
1 teaspoon sea salt

1. Trim chicken livers.
2. Broil chicken livers about 4 inches from heat, turning frequently, until brown outside and no longer pink inside, 5–10 minutes.
3. Meanwhile, in a large skillet, cook onions in butter over medium heat until golden brown, about 10 minutes.
4. Scrape onions and olive oil into a food processor.
5. Add liver, salt, and pepper and pulse until coarsely chopped. Add eggs (or egg yolks) and chop to desired consistency. Drizzle lemon juice.

Serve with French green beans and butter.

Diced Chicken   4 servings

2 cups diced cooked chicken
2 tablespoons butter
2 tablespoons soy flour
1 cup cream (diluted with water), heated
1/2 cup undiluted cream
2 tablespoons (dry) sherry
2 egg yolks, beaten
1/2 teaspoon sea salt
1/4 teaspoon white pepper
Dash of hot pepper sauce
1 pinch celery salt

1. Melt butter in a frying pan over medium heat. Stir in flour and cook about 2 minutes, stirring constantly, without browning.
2. Gradually whisk in 1 cup cream (diluted with water) and bring to a boil. Lower heat, stirring constantly, until mixture thickens. Add white pepper, sea salt, hot pepper sauce.
3. Whisk in 1/2 cup undiluted cream. Add sherry and chicken. Season with additional salt and white pepper to taste. Cook until hot. Remove from heat. Whisk in egg yolks, blending well, and serve.

Chicken Nuggets   4-6 servings

2 1/2 lb. boneless chicken breasts, cut into 1-inch pieces
Olive oil
1/2 cup cream (diluted with 1 cup spring water)
1/4 cup soy flour
1/4 cup grated Parmesan cheese
1 teaspoon paprika
1/2 teaspoon oregano

1. In a large frying pan, heat 1 inch of oil to 350°F.
2. Meanwhile, put cream in a bowl. In a paper bag, combine flour, Parmesan cheese, paprika, and oregano. Shake to mix well. First dip chicken pieces in cream; then place about a dozen pieces of chicken at a time in bag and shake until they are evenly coated.
3. Fry chicken in hot oil in batches, turning occasionally, for about 5 minutes, until crisp and golden brown. Drain on paper towels, serve hot.

"B" Ground Meat

St. Tropez Meat Roll   4-6 servings

1 1/2 pounds ground beef
1 1/2 pounds vegetables (carrots, celery, tomatoes, onions), sliced
1 egg
1 tablespoon butter (or vegetable or olive oil)
1/4 teaspoon cayenne pepper
1 pinch celery salt
1 pinch nutmeg

1. Preheat oven to 350°F.
2. In a small frying pan, combine butter and onions until lightly brown. Add vegetables; cook until tender.
3. In a small bowl, combine ground beef, egg, salt, and pepper. Mix well.
4. Press ground beef into ½-inch thickness on aluminum wrap. Place vegetables evenly over meat.
5. Roll up meat and vegetables—gently forming tube shape.
6. Place meat on baking sheet. Bake meat approximately 45 minutes. Remove from heat, cut in slices, and serve with salad.

French Cabbage Roll   4 servings

1 large white cabbage
2 pounds ground beef
1/2 pound mushrooms (optional)
2 whole eggs
1/2 cup sour cream
3 large onions, chopped
1 clove garlic, crushed through a press
4 tablespoons butter or olive oil
1 pinch thyme
1 pinch cumin
1 pinch fennel seeds
1 pinch pepper and 1 pinch sweet Hungarian (or regular) paprika
1 pinch sea salt

1. Place cabbage in a vegetable steamer (or in boiling water) until leaves are tender when pierced with tip of sharp knife. Separate tender leaves.
2. In a small frying pan, cook onions until golden brown.
3. In a big bowl, combine beef, onions, eggs, and spices. Mix well.
4. On a big plate, arrange leaves and form meat mixture into balls. Arrange beef mixture on cabbage leaves. Wrap cabbage around meat. Bind each with string or thread.
5. In a large frying pan, melt 4 tablespoons of butter over medium heat. Add onions, and cabbage rolls. Cook cabbage rolls, turning, until brown. When golden brown, add sour cream and 1/2 cup of water. Cook on low for 45 minutes. Serve warm.

Farmer's Meatballs   4-6 servings

1 pound ground beef
1 large onion, finely chopped
1 large onion, peeled and quartered
2 tablespoons soy flour
1 egg
2 cloves garlic, chopped
1 tablespoon butter
1/4 cup capers and laurels to taste
1 pinch herb salt and 1 pinch pepper
1 cup vegetable broth

1. In a large bowl, combine ground beef with egg and spices, until blended. Mix well. Form meatballs by rolling between palms of hands.
2. In medium frying pan, add 1 onion (cut in halves), laurels, garlic, and meatballs. Cook on medium heat, for 10 minutes.
3. In a medium saucepan, melt 1 tablespoon butter over medium heat, add soy flour and stir until thick. Slowly add 1 cup vegetable broth, sour cream, and capers and stir until well-blended. Simmer until a thick sauce is formed.
4. Put sauce over cooked meatballs and serve with vegetables such as green peas and carrots.

Italian Stuffed Green Peppers   4-6 servings

2 pounds ground meat
2 middle-size onions, sliced
2 middle-size onions, cut in halves
8 green peppers (or 8 zucchini or 8 large tomatoes)
5 cloves garlic, crushed through a press (or garlic powder to taste)
1/2 bunch parsley, chopped
1/2 bunch cilantro, chopped
1/2 bunch dill, chopped
2 tablespoons butter or olive oil
1 bouillon cube
Pinch saffron
Juice of 1 lemon

8. In a food processor or blender, combine parsley, cilantro, garlic, and dill with a small amount of water. Process until a puree forms.
9. In a large bowl, combine meat, eggs, vegetable puree, and seasonings (except saffron and lemon). Blend well.
10. With a sharp knife, cut off tops of green peppers. Carefully remove seeds and veins, leaving stems intact.
11. Stuff vegetable with meat mixture.
12. Preheat oven to 350°F. Place stuffed peppers in a large greased baking dish. Bake for 45 minutes to 1 hour.
13. In a small frying pan, heat 1 cup of water and add 1 bouillon cube, saffron and lemon juice. Add baking dish. Bake until peppers are tender. Remove from oven.
14. Top with sour cream. Serve warm.

Rochelle's Meatballs   4-6 servings

2 pounds ground meat
2 onions, chopped
2 onions, sliced
2 stalks celery, chopped
3–4 cloves garlic
1/2 bunch parsley
1 large can Italian peeled tomatoes, 12 ounces
Olive oil to taste
Soy flour as needed, see below
Soy sauce to taste
Sea salt to taste
Pepper to taste
Celery salt, oregano, basil to taste

1. In a food processor or blender combine chopped onions, celery, garlic, parsley, sea salt, pepper, celery salt, oregano and basil. Process vegetables. Process until a puree forms.
2. Mix vegetable puree into chop meat; mix very well; add soy flour until it is still moist but can be formed into balls by rolling mixture into 1 1/2" diameter balls in palms of hands.
3. In a frying pan, combine butter and sliced onions until lightly brown. Add salt, pepper, oregano, parsley, celery salt, and basil. Mix well. Add Italian peeled tomatoes. Chop up while cooking. Add meatballs and cook (low), turning, about 1 hour. Add soy sauce to taste.

"B" Meat

Beef with Cabbage à la Napoli 4-6 servings

3 pounds ground beef
1 large white cabbage, sliced
1 cup shredded mozzarella cheese
1 medium onion, chopped
1/2 cup olive oil
1 can (14 ounces) Italian peeled tomatoes
1 can (8 ounces) tomato sauce
1/2 cup soy flour
1 teaspoon sea salt
1 teaspoon celery salt and 1 teaspoon sea salt
2 teaspoons caraway seeds
2 apples, peeled, cored and chopped

1. In a paper or plastic bag, mix soy flour, sea salt, and caraway seeds. Add meat, a bit at a time, and shake until evenly coated.
2. In a large frying pan, heat oil over medium heat. Add meat preparation and cook, turning, until cooked. Transfer to a medium baking dish.
3. Preheat oven to 350°F. In the same pan, cook onion about 3 minutes, until tender. Add tomatoes, tomato sauce, apples, sea salt. Bring to a boil. Add cabbage and mix well. Spoon mixture over meat.
4. Cover with foil and bake 1 hour, until meat is tender. Remove foil; sprinkle mozzarella cheese over meat. Return to oven for about 5 minutes, until cheese melts.

Zurich "Geschnetzeltes"   4 servings

1 1/2 pounds beef or veal
1 pound mushrooms, sliced
1 can green peas, drained
2 cups heavy cream
Butter to taste
2 large onions, chopped
4 cloves garlic, crushed through a press
Celery salt to taste
Garlic powder to taste
Sea salt to taste
Pepper to taste

1. Cut meat in 1/2-inch slices with a sharp knife or have butcher prepare. Season with celery salt and pepper.
2. In a small frying pan, combine butter, onions and garlic until lightly brown. Add meat and cook, turning, until brown. Reduce heat and add mushrooms, spices and heavy cream. Cook, stirring occasionally, about 1 hour. Add peas and season to taste.

Cotoletta Milanese   2 servings

1/2 pound veal cutlets
8 oz. cream cheese
Butter
1 pinch nutmeg
1 pinch onion powder
1 pinch sea salt
1 pinch pepper
1 pinch celery salt
1 lemon, juice of

1. Season both sides of meat to taste.
2. In a frying pan, melt butter over medium heat. Add meat. Cook, turning, until golden brown, approximately 10 minutes. Top with lemon juice.
3. Cut cream cheese into 1/8-inch slices and arrange over meat. Allow to melt. Serve with vegetables and salad.

King Arthur's Roast with Red Cabbage) 6 servings

5–6 pound roast beef, sliced
2 large onions, sliced
5 cloves garlic, crushed through a press
4 laurels
2 cups sour (or heavy) cream
3 tablespoons olive oil
4 cups water
1 bouillon cube (vegetable, chicken, or beef)
Red wine to taste

> In a large Dutch oven, heat oil, then cook onions and garlic until brown. Add meat and red wine. Cook for 2 minutes. Add 4 cups of water and 1 bouillon cube. Cook meat, covered, occasionally stirring, until tender. Add sour (or heavy) cream. Serve with red cabbage and salad.

Austrian Meat Hodgepodge   4-6 servings

2 pounds beef, diced
1 cup water or broth (vegetable or beef)
½ cup red wine
2 large onions, sliced
2 large zucchinis, sliced
4 large carrots, sliced
1 eggplant, diced
1 clove garlic, minced
2 tomatoes, coarsely chopped
1 cup sour cream
2 bunch leeks, chopped
1 bunch cilantro, chopped
3 tablespoons butter
1/4 teaspoon sea salt
1 pinch pepper
1 pinch celery salt
1 pinch garlic powder

1. In a large Dutch oven, melt 3 tablespoons butter over medium heat.
2. Add onions and cook until golden brown, about 5 minutes. Add meat, turning, until brown.
3. Add wine and broth, vegetables and garlic.
4. Cook, covered, over medium heat. Season with sea salt and pepper to taste. Add fresh sour cream.

About "B" Grilled Dishes and Steaks

T-bone steak, sirloin steak, beef ribs, prime ribs, and any kind of grilled dishes should not be marinated with syrup or sauces containing sugar. You can marinate with natural products like lemon, vinegar, wine, cognac, garlic powder, celery salt, sea salt, or pepper or dress with soy flour, mixed with egg yolks.

T-bone steak, sirloin steak, and any other steak and grilled dishes can be served with grilled tomatoes, onions, pepper, zucchini, mushrooms, and any other vegetable (except potatoes and kale); fried eggs and sour cream with (or without) chives; herb butter; or any other dip that doesn't contain sugar (see recipes).

Hors d'oeuvres, like avocados with shrimp, are perfect. The grilled dish can be completed with "A&B Power Salad" or any other salads, fruit salad, apple dessert, or any other fruit dessert with whipped cream or ice cream (see recipes).

"B" Fish

The following dishes can be served with mixed salads, vegetables, "B" fruits and "Neutral" fruits (NO fruits from the "A" group), and all kind of cheeses. Avocados with shrimp, lemon and dill; shrimp cocktail with mayonnaise, mozzarella with tomatoes, vinegar, oil, pepper, and salt are all great hors d'oeuvres. However, for health reasons, you should eat cooked fish with (fresh) base-building foods.

Fillet of Flounder with Vegetables   2-4 servings

4 flounder fillets, about 5 ounces each
2 tablespoons butter; more if needed
2 medium carrots, cut into 1/4-inch slivers
2 ounces green beans, stemmed, stringed and cut into long, thin strips (about 2 dozen)
1/4 cup (dry) white wine or water
1/2 teaspoon salt
1/4 teaspoon pepper

1. Preheat oven to 425°F. Arrange fish flat in a single layer in a medium greased baking dish. Season with salt and pepper; set aside.
2. In a small saucepan, melt butter over very low heat. Add carrots, cover, and cook until slightly softened, 3–5 minutes. Stir in beans; cover and cook 1 minute longer. Remove cover and pour in wine. Bring to a boil.
3. Pour vegetable mixture over fish and cover dish loosely with aluminum foil. Bake 10 minutes, until fish is firm and opaque throughout.

Halibut Parmesan   4 servings

2 pounds fresh halibut steaks, cut 1 inch thick
3 tablespoons olive oil
1 medium onion, finely chopped
1 1/2 pounds fresh plum tomatoes, seeded and coarsely chopped,
OR
1 (14-ounce) can Italian peeled tomatoes, drained and chopped
2 teaspoons chopped fresh oregano or 1 teaspoon dried
1/4 teaspoon salt
1/8 teaspoon pepper
1 tablespoon tomato paste (optional)
1/2 cup grated Parmesan cheese

1. Preheat oven to 350°F.
2. Heat 2 tablespoons vegetable/olive oil in a medium saucepan. Add onion and cook until softened but not brown, 3–5 minutes. Stir in tomatoes and season with oregano, salt, and pepper. Stir in tomato paste for a deeper flavor, if desired. Reduce heat to medium-low and simmer, stirring frequently, until sauce is slightly thickened, about 10 minutes. Let cool slightly; then transfer to a food processor. Puree until smooth.
3. Pour tomato sauce into baking dish. Arrange fish on top. Grate Parmesan cheese and sprinkle evenly over fish.
4. Bake 15 minutes until fish is opaque throughout. Serve at once.

Baked Whitefish with Tomato   2-4 servings

1 pound whitefish fillets
1 cup celery stalks, chopped
2 small carrots, chopped
1 (28-ounce) can Italian peeled tomatoes, drained and coarsely chopped
1 medium onion, chopped
2 tablespoons olive oil
2 pounds fresh spinach
1/2 plus 1/8 teaspoon salt and 1/4 teaspoon pepper

1. Preheat oven to 350°F.
2. In a large saucepan, combine carrots, onion, and celery. Stir in olive oil and cook over medium heat until vegetables are softened, 5–7 minutes. Add tomatoes, 1/2 teaspoon salt, and

pepper. Cook over medium heat, stirring occasionally, until thick and pulpy, about 10 minutes. Transfer to a food processor and puree tomato sauce until smooth.

3. If using fresh spinach, plunge leaves in a large pot of rapidly boiling salted water. Return to a boil and immediately drain. Rinse under cold running water. If using frozen spinach, cook according to package directions. Use your hands to squeeze out excess moisture from spinach; coarsely chop.

4. Spread chopped spinach over bottom of a buttered medium baking dish. Cut whitefish crosswise into 1/2-inch-thick slices. Layer over spinach and season with remaining 1/8 teaspoon salt. Spread tomato sauce over fish. Cover dish loosely with aluminum foil. Bake 10 minutes, or until sauce is bubbly and fish is firm and white. Serve at once.

Baked Sole with Orange   4 servings

1 1/2 pounds sole fillets
1/2 teaspoon salt
1/4 teaspoon pepper
1/4 cup fresh orange juice
1 teaspoon soy flour
1/4 cup fresh lemon juice
1 whole orange

1. Arrange fish in a baking dish large enough to hold fillets flat in a single layer. Season with salt and pepper. Add orange juice and lemon juice. Cover and refrigerate 1 hour.

2. Use a serrated knife to cut away peel from orange. Cut between membranes to remove whole sections. Place in a small bowl and set aside.

3. Preheat oven to 350°F. Remove fish from refrigerator and cover dish tightly with aluminum foil. Bake 8–10 minutes, until firm and opaque throughout.

4. Transfer fillets to warm serving plates. Pour cooking liquid into a small saucepan. Dissolve soy flour in 2 tablespoons cold water. Stir into liquid in saucepan and bring to a boil over medium-high heat, stirring until thickened, for 1 minute. Add more soy flour as needed. Spread sauce over fillets; garnish with orange slices.

Sole Meuniere   4 servings

4 sole fillets, 4 to 6 ounces each
1/2 cup soy flour
1/2 cup cream diluted with a little water
4 tablespoons butter
½ cup olive oil
2 tablespoons chopped parsley
1/2 teaspoon salt
1/4 teaspoon pepper
1 tablespoon fresh lemon

1. In a shallow bowl, combine soy flour, salt, and pepper. Dip sole in diluted cream, then dredge in soy flour mixture to coat.
2. In a large skillet, heat oil over medium-high heat until bubbling. Shake excess soy flour off dredged fish and arrange fish in pan. Cook, turning once, until brown and crisp, about 2 minutes each side. Remove to serving plates. Drain off fat from pan.
3. Return skillet to heat and add 4 tablespoons of butter, parsley, and lemon juice. Stir until butter is melted and well blended. Spoon a small amount of sauce over each fillet and serve.

Wolfish (Loup De Mere) with Mushrooms 4 servings

1 1/2 pounds wolfish fillets, or other fish fillets, cut into 4 equal pieces
1 clove garlic, minced
2 tablespoons butter
2 bunches scallions, chopped
1/4 pound mushrooms, thinly sliced
1 (28-ounce) can Italian peeled tomatoes, drained and chopped
10 large cabbage leaves, chopped
1/2 teaspoon salt
1/4 teaspoon pepper

1. Cut tough rib ends from cabbage leaves. Bring a large pot of salted water to boil over high heat. Add cabbage leaves and boil until limp, 3 to 5 minutes. Drain and rinse under cold running water; drain again. Lay flat on paper towels and pat dry.

2. In a large saucepan, melt butter over medium-high heat. Add scallions and garlic. Cook, stirring, until slightly softened, about 1 minute. Add mushrooms and tomatoes. Increase heat to high and boil, stirring often, until sauce is slightly thickened, about 3 minutes. Season with salt and pepper and set aside

3. Preheat oven to 425°F. Place 3 cabbage leaves together on a work surface, stem ends overlapping in center. Place a piece of fish in center. Season lightly with additional salt and pepper. Bring up ends and sides, envelope fashion, to completely cover the fish. Continue with remaining leaves and fish. Carefully transfer each to a buttered medium baking dish, placing each bundle snugly next to the other, seam side down.

4. Spread tomato-mushroom mixture over fish. Cover dish loosely with aluminum foil. Bake 10–12 minutes, or until fish is firm and sauce is bubbly.

Swordfish Steaks   4 servings

4 swordfish steaks, 4 to 6 ounces each
2 tablespoons grated Parmesan cheese
2 cloves garlic, peeled
1/3 cup olive oil
1/4 cup pine nuts
1 cup fresh basil leaves
1/4 teaspoon salt
1/8 teaspoon pepper
Lemon slices

1. Preheat oven to 425°F. Arrange fish steaks in a large, lightly oiled baking dish. In a food processor, combine basil, garlic, pine nuts, Parmesan cheese, salt, and pepper. Puree until smooth. With machine on, slowly pour in olive oil. Process until mixture is well blended.

2. Spread mixture evenly over swordfish steaks. Cover dish loosely with aluminum foil. Bake until steaks are white throughout but still moist, 10–12 minutes. Garnish with thin slices of lemon.

Swordfish (or Tuna)   4 servings

4 (1-inch-thick) swordfish (or tuna) steaks, about 6 ounces each
2 medium ripe tomatoes, peeled, seeded, and chopped
2 tablespoons vegetable or olive oil
1 small clove garlic, crushed through a press
1/2 teaspoon salt
1/4 teaspoon pepper
1 tablespoon dried thyme
1/4 cup dry white wine

1. In a large frying pan, cook swordfish (or tuna) in vegetable or olive oil over medium-high heat, turning once, 7–9 minutes. Remove to a serving platter and cover with aluminum foil to keep warm.
2. Pour off fat in pan. Add white wine, increase heat to high, and boil, stirring constantly, until reduced by half, about 1 minute. Stir in tomatoes, thyme, and garlic. Reduce heat to medium and cook, stirring often, until thick and pulpy, 3–5 minutes. Season with salt and pepper. Spoon tomato sauce over swordfish or tuna and serve.

Smoked Salmon and Parmesan   2 servings

3 ounces thinly sliced smoked salmon
1/4 teaspoon hot pepper sauce
Dash of lemon juice
8 ounces natural cream cheese, softened
1 cup fresh dill or parsley
3/4 cup grated Parmesan cheese (about 3 ounces)

1. Preheat oven to 400°F. In a small bowl or food processor, combine cream cheese, Parmesan cheese, lemon juice, and hot sauce. Blend well.
2. Cut smoked salmon into 30 pieces. Spoon about 2 teaspoons of cheese mixture over salmon and top each with dill (or parsley). Bake in greased baking dish until cheese is just softened, about 5 minutes. Serve warm.

Butter-Fried Shrimp   4 servings

1 1/2 pounds large shrimp
1 1/2 cups soy flour
2 tablespoons butter, melted and cooled
2 eggs, separated
1 cup olive oil
8 broccoli florets
1 small onion, sliced
1 teaspoon salt
1/2 teaspoon pepper

1. Slit shrimp down back and remove intestinal vein and shell; leave tails intact. Spread shrimp open to butterfly. Keep refrigerated until ready to cook.
2. In a large mixing bowl, combine soy flour, butter, salt, pepper, and egg yolks. Mix to form a thin batter. Cover and refrigerate for 4–6 hours.
3. When ready to cook, preheat oven to 200°F. Pour enough olive oil into a deep-fat fryer or large frying pan. Heat to 375°F. Beat egg whites until stiff and fold into batter. In batches, without crowding, dip shrimp into batter, one at a time, and drop into hot olive oil. Fry until lightly brown, 3 minutes. Drain on paper towels and keep warm in oven while frying vegetables.
4. Dip onion slices and broccoli florets into batter, one at a time, and fry for 1 to 1-1/2 minutes, or until coating is crisp and light beige in color. Drain on paper towels, transfer to oven to keep warm.
5. Serve shrimp with vegetables.

"B" Soups

Chicken Soup   4-6 servings

5 pounds stewing chicken, cut up
6 cups (filtered) water
3 stalks celery, cut up
1 small onion, cut up
1/4 teaspoon salt
1/8 teaspoon pepper
1 bay leaf
16 ounces Italian peeled tomatoes (can), cut up
3 medium carrots, cut into julienne strips
1/2 cup onions, chopped
4 teaspoons instant chicken bouillon granules (sold in a jar)
1 cup zucchini, halved lengthwise and sliced

1. In a large Dutch oven, combine chicken pieces, water, onion, celery, salt, pepper, and bay leaf. Bring to a boil. Reduce heat and simmer, covered, for 2 hours until chicken is tender. Remove chicken from broth. Let stand until chicken is cool enough to handle; then cut off meat and cube chicken; set aside.
2. Meanwhile, strain broth, discarding vegetables and bay leaf. Return broth to stove. Stir in tomatoes, onion, carrots, and bouillon. Simmer, covered, for 20 minutes until carrots are almost tender.
3. Add chicken to broth mixture along with zucchini. Simmer, covered, about 5 minutes until vegetables are tender.

"B" Vegetables

Eggplant with Tomatoes   4-6 servings

2 large eggplants (or 4 small)
6 cloves garlic, crushed through a press
2 medium tomatoes, pureed
4 small onions, peeled
1 cup olive oil
1 bunch parsley, chopped
1 bunch cilantro, chopped
Sea salt
Pepper
Celery salt

1. With a sharp knife, remove stem end of eggplants. Cut eggplants in 1/2-inch slices; salt and drain liquid onto paper towels.
2. Chop cilantro and parsley. Puree tomatoes. Add garlic. Mix well.
3. In a large frying pan, heat cooking oil. Place eggplants in oil. Fry until brown. Pat off oil with paper towels.
4. Preheat oven to 300°F. On a baking sheet, place eggplants. Sprinkle tomato-cilantro-parsley mixture over eggplants. Bake for 20 minutes, until crispy. Season to taste.

"B" Salads

Waldorf Astoria Salad

2 cups diced apples (2 medium apples)
2 sweet oranges, diced (without seeds)
1 pound cooked chicken, diced
3/4 cup celery, coarsely chopped
1 cup mayonnaise
1 cup sour cream
4 tablespoons heavy cream, whipped
1/2 cup coarsely chopped walnuts
1 dash cognac
2 tablespoons lemon juice (or vinegar)
1 dash salt

> In medium bowl, combine all ingredients (except whipped cream, sour cream, and walnuts). Mix well. Chill thoroughly. Add whipped cream, sour cream, and walnuts before serving. Serve on lettuce. Refrigerate leftovers.

Hawaiian Chicken Salad

1/2 pound cooked chicken (or leftovers), diced
2 cups pineapple, diced
1 cup mayonnaise
Dash vinegar
Dash pepper
Pinch garlic salt
Pinch nutmeg

> In medium bowl, combine all ingredients except pineapples; mix well. Chill thoroughly. Serve on lettuce; top with diced pineapple.

Peking Chicken Salad

1 pound cooked chicken (or any kind of poultry), diced
2 oranges, diced (without seeds)
1 peel of orange, grated
2 cups mayonnaise
1 cup almonds, cut in halves
Dash cognac
Pinch nutmeg

In a large bowl, combine all ingredients; mix well. Chill thoroughly. Serve on lettuce; garnish with orange slices.

Carrot Salad d'Alsace

4 large carrots
1/4 pound cooked ham, cut into thing ¼" slivers
Juice of 2 oranges
1 peel of orange, grated
2 cups mayonnaise
Dash garlic powder
Dash pepper
Dash nutmeg

Cut carrots into 1/8-inch slices. Combine ham, with juice of grated oranges and grated peel of oranges; add mayonnaise. Mix well. Add to carrots. Chill thoroughly. Serve on lettuce.

Swiss Cheese Salad

1/2 pound Swiss cheese, thinly sliced
2 medium onions, thinly sliced into rings
Olive oil to taste
Vinegar to taste
Salt to taste
Pepper to taste

In medium bowl, combine all ingredients. Add salt and pepper to taste. Mix well.

Sylvia's Tuna Salad

1 (6 1/2 ounce) can tuna (in oil or water)
1/4 cup capers, either small capers or halve large ones
3 tablespoons onion, chopped
2 tablespoons mustard
1/2 cup pickled cucumbers, diced
1/3 cup parsley, chopped
Olive oil, quantity to taste
1 teaspoon fresh lemon juice (or vinegar)
1/4 teaspoon pepper
Salt to taste
Garlic salt to taste

In a medium bowl, drain then mash tuna with oil and mustard. Add onions, lemon juice, pickled cucumber dices, ½ the capers, salt and pepper. Mix well. Serve on lettuce. Garnish with remaining pickled cucumber slices.

Bavarian Sausage Salad

1/2 pound Bologna sausage, sliced
2 medium onions, thinly sliced into rings
Olive oil to taste
Vinegar to taste
Salt to taste
Pepper to taste

1. Cut across sausage in 1/4-inch slices.
2. Mix with onion slices.
3. Add oil, vinegar, salt and pepper. Mix well.

Chef Salad

Lettuce (quantity to taste)
Tomatoes, sliced or diced into cubes
Cucumber, thinly sliced
Broccoli, sliced
Cauliflower, sliced
Carrots, thinly sliced
Onions, sliced or diced into cubes
1–2 boiled eggs, sliced
Swiss cheese, thinly sliced
Smoked ham, sliced
Cooked turkey or chicken, lenghtwise sliced
Oil to taste
Vinegar to taste
Salt to taste
Pepper to taste
Mayonnaise (OPTIONAL: dip or dressing)

1. Cut up vegetables. In a large bowl, combine all vegetables, smoked ham, and turkey or chicken.
2. Add oil, vinegar, salt, and pepper. Add mayonnaise (or dip or dressing). Mix well.

"B" Hors d'Oeuvre

Avocados with Shrimp   1–2 servings

1 large avocado (1/2 for every person)
1 can shrimp, drained
4 tablespoons lemon juice
1 bunch dill, chopped
4 tablespoons olive oil
Salt to taste
Pepper to taste

1. Using a sharp knife, cut avocado in half. Remove pit.
2. In a medium bowl, combine lemon juice, oil, salt, and pepper to taste. Mix well.
3. Arrange shrimp on avocado. Top with dill. Pour liquid mixture over avocado and dill. Serve immediately or cover with plastic wrap to prevent avocado from darkening. Refrigerate.

"B" Desserts

Creamy Fruit Dessert

1 pound strawberries, chopped
1 pound raspberries, chopped
1/2 pound peaches, chopped
2 cups heavy cream, whipped
Sweetener

Mix ingredients well and refrigerate until ready to eat.

Apple Dessert

5 medium apples, cored, peeled, and 1/2-inch sliced
Olive oil
Dash cinnamon powder

In a frying pan, heat oil and fry 1/2-inch apple slices until golden
brown. Sprinkle cinnamon powder to taste. Eat warm or cold.

Baked Apple

5 apples, peeled
1/2 cup walnuts, coarse-grained, chopped
Sweetener

1. Remove cores from apples. Fill apples with walnuts.
2. Preheat oven to 350°F. Top every apple with a piece of butter
    and sweetener.. Bake until lightly browned.

413

Swiss Fruit Salad

1 grapefruit, diced
2 sweet oranges, diced
2 apples, cored, peeled, and sliced in cubes
1 cup pineapple, diced
1 peel of orange, grated
2 cups whipped cream, chilled
1 dash cognac
1 dash cinnamon
Sweetener

In a large bowl, combine all ingredients. Refrigerate for 30 minutes. Serve cold.

"B" Ice Cream

Strawberry Ice Cream
(Or any other "B" fruit, such as raspberries or kiwis)

2 cups heavy cream, whipped
1 pound fruit

1. In a processor, combine whipped cream with fruit.
2. In a plastic bowl, put mixture into freezer and chill at least for 1–1 1/2 hours. Serve with whipped cream. Garnish with fresh fruits.

"Neutral" Recipes

"Neutral" Breakfast

The best breakfast is indeed milk (or yogurt) with apples, because you will build a strong alkaline foundation for the day. However, if you would like to eat other tasty "Neutral" breakfasts try these:

- Blueberries with yogurt, blueberries with cream or whipped cream

- Goat's milk cheese or sheep's milk cheese, Camembert, or any other cream cheese with vegetables, salads, and/or sprouts

- Cottage cheese or ricotta cheese with apples or any other "B" or Neutral fruit

- Cottage cheese or ricotta cheese, mixed with cream and herbs

- Smoked ham, smoked sausages, salami, beef-salami, bacon, rolled ham, or any cured, dried, or smoked meat with vegetables and/or salads

- Smoked herring, smoked mackerel, smoked salmon, or any smoked fish with vegetables and/or salads and/or dips

"Neutral" Lunches and Dinners

"Neutral" Beans

Beans are believed to be difficult to digest, yet fava beans are the Egyptian national dish. The Egyptians <u>don't have any problem digesting beans</u>. They soak the beans for several hours in water to prepare them (unknowingly) for a chemical process that makes digestion easier. The Egyptians eat fava beans with wheat bread, olive oil, and several raw onions, radishes, and/or special salads (Ramses Salad), which are base-builders.

Ramses Beans with Ramses Salad

Old Egyptian recipe; beans should be eaten with Ramses Salad (or raw onions) to ensure proper digestion.

2 pounds small fava beans
1 pound skinless fava beans
1 pound garbanzo beans (chickpeas)
1/2 pound yellow lentils
1 large garlic bulb, crushed through a press
2 tablespoon cumin
2 tablespoon dried coriander
Salt to taste
Pepper to taste

1. Wash beans and lentils separately. In a big bowl, combine fava beans, skinless fava beans, and garbanzo beans. Cover beans with plenty of (distilled) cold water. Soak beans for 3–4 hours, <u>preferably longer</u>. Remove from water.
2. In a large saucepan, bring water to a boil. Add fava beans and garbanzo beans. Cover with water, 4 inches above. Reduce heat.
3. Check the water level every hour; add water if necessary.
4. Simmer over medium-low heat for 4–5 hours, until soft. As soon as beans are soft, add lentils. Let cook, for 1 hour, until soft. Add garlic, cumin, coriander, salt, and pepper. Let stand, for 30 minutes. Serve warm; top the Ramses Beans with Ramses Salad.

(OPTIONAL: mash beans with mixer. Top beans with Ramses Salad.)

Ramses Salad

(OPTIONAL: Onions, dressed with vinegar, pepper, salt, and cumin. Crush onions with your hand to enhance flavor.)

5–6 fresh hot peppers, such as jalapenos
2–3 large tomatoes
2 large onions
1 head lettuce
1 bunch cilantro
6 large cloves garlic
1 tablespoon coriander
1 tablespoon cumin
Salt to taste
Pepper to taste
1/2 cup vinegar
1/2 cup olive oil

> Combine all ingredients in a food processor. Process until well blended to form a pulp. Top Ramses Beans with 3 tablespoons Ramses Salad.

TIP: Put remaining Ramses Salad in a jar. Cover with olive oil, 2 inches above pulp. Refrigerate for later use. (Also tastes great as a dip with whole wheat bread or pita.)

"Neutral" Soups

Oriental Lentil Soup   4-6 servings

1 1/2 cups lentils, dried
2 cups vegetable or 2 chicken bouillon (cubes in 2 cups water)
8 cups spring water
1 large onion, minced
1 clove garlic, crushed through a press
2 stalks celery, chopped
2 large carrots, chopped
2 tablespoons fresh parsley, chopped
1/2 teaspoon dried thyme
1/2 teaspoon sea salt
3 tablespoons olive oil
1 teaspoon dried oregano
1 teaspoon sweet Hungarian (or regular) paprika

1. In a saucepan, heat oil over medium-high setting. Add onions, tossing for 5 minutes, until crisp-tender.
2. Add garlic, carrots and celery. Add seasoning and herbs; mix well, tossing for 3–4 minutes.
3. Add vegetable or chicken bouillon; cook for 3 minutes.
4. Add lentils and 8 cups water. Simmer over low heat for about 60 minutes; add parsley.

Creamy Cauliflower Soup   4-6 servings

6 cups spring water
2 medium cauliflowers, cored and coarsely chopped
1 onion, chopped
1 clove garlic, crushed through a press
2 tablespoons butter
1 tablespoon olive oil
2 stalks celery, chopped
8 scallions, chopped
2 tablespoons vegetable bouillon (or broth)
1/8 teaspoon fresh ground black pepper
1/8 teaspoon nutmeg
1 teaspoon dried basil
1/2 teaspoon dried thyme
1 teaspoon dried marjoram
1/2 teaspoon celery or sea salt

In a large saucepan, melt butter and heat oil. Add scallions, onions, garlic, cauliflower and celery. Season with salt and pepper to taste. Cook over medium heat for several minutes, stirring frequently. Add broth or bouillon; bring to a boil. Add basil, thyme and marjoram. Simmer, covered, over medium heat until cauliflower is tender, for 10–15 minutes. Remove cover and cool slightly. In blender, process until soup is smooth and creamy. Repeat; add nutmeg to taste.

"Neutral" Vegetables

Broccoli Milanese   2 servings

4 stalks broccoli, washed and stems cut off
2 tablespoons butter
2 teaspoons fresh lemon juice or vinegar
Seasoning to taste

1. Cut broccoli into individual florets. Place in vegetable steamer over boiling water until tender, covered, for 7 minutes.
2. In small saucepan, melt butter; combine with lemon juice. Pour sauce over hot broccoli. Season to taste.

Carrots Vienna   4 servings

12 medium carrots, peeled
3 tablespoons butter
1/4 teaspoon sea salt
2 teaspoons fresh (or dried) basil
Soy sauce

1. Cut carrots into 1/8-inch slices. Place carrots in a vegetable steamer over boiling water until tender, for 5-8 minutes. Remove from heat and set aside.
2. In large saucepan, melt butter. Add carrots, basil and sea salt. Stir well. Season to taste.

Mushrooms Lyon   2 servings

1/2 pound mushrooms
1 tablespoon butter
1 tablespoon fresh lemon juice
Dash sea salt
Dash garlic powder
Soy sauce

1. Wash mushrooms; cut ends from stems. Cut mushrooms into slices.
2. In a saucepan, melt butter. Add mushrooms, tossing lightly in butter, until soft. Add lemon juice. Season to taste with sea salt or soy sauce.

Vegetables Parisian   4 servings

6 peeled carrots, cut into cubes
2 medium zucchini, sliced
2 medium yellow squash
2 tablespoons butter
2 teaspoons fresh lemon juice or vinegar
Soy sauce to taste
Seasoning to taste

1. In a vegetable steamer, place carrots over boiling water for 10 minutes. Add zucchini and steam until tender, for 7 minutes.
2. Arrange vegetables on a plate. Cut squash in cubes. Combine butter and lemon juice (or vinegar) and pour over vegetables. Season to taste.

Artichokes Venetian

4 servings

4 artichokes
Several celery stalks
1 bay leaf
1 clove garlic, crushed through a press

1. Wash artichokes. Trim end of stem. Snip thorny tip off each leaf. Combine garlic, celery stalks, and bay leaf.
2. In a vegetable steamer, place artichokes over boiling water, for 30–40 minutes, according to size. As soon as leaves can be removed, discard bay leaf, celery, and garlic. Serve with melted butter.

Cauliflower Soufflé Côte d'Azur

4 servings

1 large cauliflower, cored and broken into small florets
3 tablespoons olive oil
2 egg yolks
1/4 cup parsley, chopped
1 pinch sweet Hungarian (or regular) paprika
1 pinch nutmeg

1. Preheat oven to 350°F.
2. In a saucepan, cook cauliflower in boiling salted water until just tender, for 10 minutes. Remove from heat.
3. Whisk two egg yolks, with 2 teaspoons oil, nutmeg, pepper, and parsley.
4. Transfer cauliflower to soufflé dish with oil.
5. Spread egg mixture over cauliflower. Place in a broiler until soufflé is golden brown, 5–7 minutes.

Eggplant Normandy   4-6 servings

2 large eggplants (or 4 small)
6 cloves garlic, crushed through a press
4 small onions, peeled
2 medium tomatoes, pureed
2 cups olive oil
1 bunch parsley, chopped
1 bunch cilantro, chopped
Sea salt
Pepper
Celery salt

1. Preheat oven to 300°F.
2. With a sharp knife, remove stem end of eggplants. Cut eggplants in 1/2-inch slices, salt and lay on paper towels to drain liquid.
3. Chop cilantro and parsley. Add garlic. Mix well.
4. In a large saucepan, heat cooking oil. Place eggplant in olive oil. Fry until brown.
5. On a baking sheet, place eggplant slices. Sprinkle tomato-cilantro-parsley mixture over eggplants. Bake for 20 minutes, until crispy. Season to taste.

Cabbage Budapest   2–3 servings

1 white cabbage, sliced
1 pound onions, diced
2 cups vegetable broth (or 2 cups water/2 bouillon cubes)
2 cups heavy cream
2 tablespoons butter
1 cup sour cream
Sea salt to taste
2 teaspoons Hungarian (or regular) paprika
Soy sauce to taste

4. In a large saucepan, sauté onions in butter until golden brown. Add vegetable broth or bouillon.
5. Place cabbage in saucepan and cook for 15–20 minutes. Remove from heat and drain cabbage.
6. Combine heavy cream with paprika and season to taste. Sprinkle mixture over cabbage. Let stand 10 minutes.

"Neutral"
Hors d'Oeuvres

Mozzarella with Tomatoes   2 servings

2 large tomatoes, sliced
1 ball mozzarella, sliced
Fresh basil
Vinegar to taste
Olive oil to taste
Salt to taste
Pepper to taste

1. Cut tomatoes and mozzarella in thin slices. Arrange on a platter or serving plate.
2. In a small bowl, combine vinegar and oil. Pour mixture over mozzarella and tomatoes. Add salt and pepper to taste. Garnish with fresh basil.

Avocados with Lemon and Olive Oil   1–2 servings

1 large avocado (1/2 for every person)
4 tablespoons lemon juice
1 bunch dill, chopped
4 tablespoons olive oil
Salt to taste
Pepper to taste

1. Using a sharp knife, cut avocado in halves. Remove pit.
2. In a medium bowl, combine lemon juice, oil, salt, and pepper to taste. Mix well.
3. Top with dill. Pour mixture over avocado and dill. Serve immediately, or cover with plastic wrap to prevent avocado from darkening. Refrigerate.

OPTIONAL: Dill Dip or Creamy Avocado Dressing (see recipe "Salad Dressings & Other Dips")

"Neutral" Salads

There is no limit to the quantity of vegetables, salads, sprouts, and herbs you can eat. Variety is important! The best vegetables to use for the purpose of detoxification are the root vegetables—carrots, turnips, and beets—and all sorts of top vegetables, such as spinach, beet tops, chard, celery, onion tops, watercress, broccoli, cauliflower, sprouts, or any green vegetable that contains juice.

A&B Power Salad

Lettuce (romaine, iceberg, limestone, red leaf, watercress, or any other lettuce, broken into bite-size pieces)
Tomatoes, sliced or diced into cubes
Cucumber, sliced or diced into cubes
Carrots, chopped or sliced
Cauliflower, chopped
Broccoli, chopped
White and/or red cabbage, chopped
Sprouts/soy sprouts
Spinach, chopped
Onions, sliced or diced into cubes
Scallions, sliced
Parsley, chopped
Chives, chopped
Oil to taste (olive, flaxseed, sesame, etc.)
Apple vinegar (opt: Balsamic) or fresh lemon juice to taste
Salt (sea salt, herb salt, Bio-salt) to taste
Pepper to taste

1. Cut up vegetables. In a large bowl, combine all vegetables.
2. In a small bowl, combine oil, vinegar, salt, pepper, and chives.

OPTIONAL: salad dressing, chunky blue cheese dressing, mayonnaise or dip/dressing, see section "Mayonnaise, Salad Dressing and Other Dips." Pour over salad.

Classic Green Salad

1 head lettuce—butter, red leaf, iceberg, or romaine
  (washed, dried, and sliced into bite-sized pieces)
1 small cucumber, peeled and sliced
2 tomatoes, sliced
3 carrots, sliced
1 large onion, sliced
2 garlic cloves, crushed through a press
3 tablespoons olive oil
1 tablespoon fresh lemon juice or vinegar
1/4–1/2 teaspoon sea salt
1/2 teaspoon celery salt

> Place all ingredients in a bowl. Pour dressing over salad and toss well.

Ramses Salad

5–6 fresh hot peppers, such as jalapenos
2 large tomatoes
2 large onions
1 head lettuce
6 cloves garlic
1/2 cup vinegar
1/2 cup olive oil
1 tablespoon coriander
1 bunch cilantro
1 tablespoon cumin
Salt to taste
Pepper to taste

> In a food processor, combine peppers, tomatoes, onions, lettuce, garlic, salt, pepper, vinegar, oil, and herbs. Process until well blended. Ideal with fava beans (see recipe "Ramses Beans"), whole wheat bread, or steamed potatoes.

Asparagus Salad

1 head lettuce
1/2 head red leaf lettuce
1/2 pound fresh (or canned) asparagus
3 tablespoons olive oil
1 tablespoon vinegar
Lemon juice to taste
1/2 teaspoon mustard
1 clove garlic, crushed through a press
Sea salt to taste
Fresh ground black pepper

1. Wash lettuce; dry and break into pieces. Break and discard heavy ends from asparagus.
2. In a medium saucepan, cook asparagus and salt in boiling salted water until tender, 3–5 minutes. Remove from water. Drain well. Cut into 1 1/2-inch pieces. Combine with lettuce.
3. For dressing, combine oil, mustard, sea salt, and lemon juice (and/or vinegar). Add pepper to taste. Mix well. Pour over salad.

Celery Salad

1 medium bunch of celery
1/2 cup mayonnaise
2 tablespoons fresh lemon juice or vinegar
2 teaspoons mustard
Seasoning to taste

1. Cut celery into very thin slices. Cut peel from slices; then julienne each slice. Add lemon juice.
2. Place celery in boiling water for 3–5 minutes until tender. Drain well.
3. Combine mayonnaise and mustard. Toss celery in mixture. Season to taste. Serve at room temperature.

Carrot Salad

1 pound large peeled carrots
Olive oil to taste
Lemon (or vinegar) to taste
Dash garlic powder
Dash pepper
Dash artificial sweetener

Slice carrots into 1/8-inch slices and put in food processor with. remaining ingredients. Mix well. Serve on lettuce.

Cucumber with Dill

4 cucumbers, peeled and sliced
1 cup sour cream
2 tablespoons fresh lemon juice or apple vinegar
2 tablespoons fresh dill, chopped, or 1 tablespoon dried dill
1/4 teaspoon sea salt
1 teaspoon scallions, minced

Combine ingredients. Mix well. Chill.

"Neutral" Desserts

Creamy Walnut Dessert

1 cup cottage cheese (or Ricotta cheese)
1/2 cup heavy cream, whipped
2 egg yolks*
1/4 cup walnuts

In a medium bowl, put ½ of walnuts and all ingredients. Mix well. Refrigerate. Top with remaining walnuts when serving.

Creamy Blueberry Dessert

2 pounds blueberries
2 cups heavy cream, whipped
Sweetener

Mix ingredients well. Refrigerate.

There is some danger of salmonella from uncooked egg yolks.

"Neutral" Ice Cream

Vanilla Ice Cream

2 cups heavy cream, whipped
4 egg yolks *
1 teaspoon vanilla
1 cup chopped walnuts
Artificial sweetener

1. In a processor, combine whipped cream with egg yolks, vanilla, and artificial sweetener. Process until mixture is foaming.
2. Put mixture into a plastic bowl. Put in freezer. Chill at least 1 to 1 1/2 hours. Serve with whipped cream. Garnish with walnuts.

Hazelnut Ice Cream

2 cups heavy cream, whipped
4 egg yolks*
2 cups hazelnuts, crushed
2 packets artificial sweetener

1. In a processor, combine whipped cream with egg yolks, hazelnuts, and artificial sweetener. Process until mixture is foaming.
2. Put mixture into plastic bowl. Put in freezer. Chill at least 1 to 1 1/2 hours. Serve with whipped cream. Garnish with hazelnuts.

* *There is some danger of salmonella from uncooked egg yolks.*

"Neutral" Mayonnaise, Salad Dresssings And Other Dips

A&B Dressing

1 cup mayonnaise
2 tablespoons horseradish

> In a bowl, combine mayonnaise and horseradish. Stir until well blended. Chill.

Classic Mayonnaise

2 egg yolks *
2 tablespoons olive oil
1 lemon juice or vinegar
Salt to taste

> In a bowl, combine refrigerated ingredients. Add drop by drop 2 tablespoons olive oil and lemon juice (or vinegar). Whisk until well blended. Refrigerate until firm.

For larger quantities user 4 egg yolks, 8 tablespoons olive oil, juice of 2 lemons, sea salt, and 5 tablespoons water. There is some danger of salmonella from uncooked egg yolks.

French Garlic Mayonnaise

5 egg yolks *
5 tablespoon olive oil
5 tablespoon (filtered) water
1 lemon juice or vinegar
6 clove of garlic, crushed through a press
Salt to taste

> Combine refrigerated ingredients. Add 5 tablespoons oil and lemon juice drop by drop. Add garlic and salt to taste. Whisk until well blended. Refrigerate until firm.

Chili Mayonnaise

1/2 cup mayonnaise
2 teaspoons chili powder
1 teaspoon ground cumin
2 teaspoons fresh lemon juice or vinegar
Dash salt
1/8 teaspoon cayenne pepper

> In a small bowl, combine ingredients, except mayonnaise. Stir until well blended. Blend in mayonnaise.

For a larger quantity use 4 egg yolks, 8 tablespoons olive oil, juice of 2 lemons, sea salt, and 5 tablespoons water. There is some danger of salmonella from uncooked egg yolks.

French Spicy Mayonnaise

1 cup mayonnaise
1 hard-boiled egg yolk, mashed
1 tablespoon chopped anchovies
1 tablespoon chopped parsley
1 tablespoon drained capers
1 teaspoon mustard
Dash cayenne pepper

>   In a small bowl, combine all ingredients. Stir until well blended. Cover and refrigerate.

Oriental Curry-Lemon Mayonnaise

1/2 cup mayonnaise
1/2 cup sour cream
1 1/2 teaspoons curry powder
1 tablespoon fresh lemon juice or vinegar
Dash salt
Dash cayenne pepper

1. In a small bowl, combine mayonnaise and sour cream. Mix until well blended. Stir in lemon juice, salt, and cayenne. Add curry powder.
2. Cover and refrigerate.

Creamy Avocado Dressing

1 avocado
1 clove garlic, crushed through a press
2 teaspoons olive oil
1/4 cup water
2 tablespoons sour cream
1 tablespoon fresh (or dried) dill
1/2 teaspoon sea salt
2 tablespoons lemon juice (or vinegar)

1. Peel avocado. Cut into large quarters.
2. Place ingredients in food processor. Process until creamy.

Dill Dip

1/2 cup mayonnaise
1/2 cup sour cream
2 tablespoons minced fresh dill (or 1 tablespoon dried dill)
2 tablespoons chopped parsley
2 tablespoons chopped scallions
1/2 teaspoon lemon juice or vinegar
1/2 teaspoon salt
1/2 teaspoon black pepper

In a small bowl, combine all ingredients. Stir until well blended. Refrigerate.

Cream Cheese Dip

2 8-ounce packages cream cheese, softened
1 scallion, minced
1 large clove garlic, crushed through a press
1 dash cayenne pepper
1 dash salt
1 dash vinegar or lemon juice
1/2 teaspoon dried dill
1/2 teaspoon dried basil
1/2 teaspoon dried marjoram
1/2 teaspoon dried thyme
1/2 teaspoon dried tarragon

In a medium bowl, combine all ingredients. Stir until well blended. Cover and refrigerate.

Chutney Cheese Spread

1 8-ounce package cream cheese
2 cups shredded sharp Cheddar cheese (about 8 ounces)
2 tablespoons dry sherry
1/2 cup mango chutney, chopped
1/4 cup scallions, chopped
1 teaspoon curry powder
1/4 teaspoon salt
Dash hot pepper sauce or cayenne pepper

1. In a saucepan combine cream cheese, Cheddar cheese, curry powder, salt, hot sauce, and sherry. Melt over low heat until smooth and well blended.
2. Cover and refrigerate until firm, about 2 hours.
3. Spread on wheat bread or pitas topped with chutney and scallions.

Horseradish Sauce

1 cup sour cream
1/3 cup horseradish
1 tablespoon fresh lemon juice or vinegar
Pinch white pepper

In a small bowl, combine all ingredients. Stir until well blended. Cover and refrigerate 1 hour.

Blue Cheese Dip

1 cup crumbled blue cheese (4 ounces)
1 tablespoon white vinegar
1 scallion, chopped
1/2 cup mayonnaise
1/2 cup sour cream
1 clove garlic, crushed through a press

1. In a small bowl, mash cheese and add all ingredients.
2. Stir until well blended.
3. Cover and refrigerate.

APPENDIX I

IMPORTANT CASE STUDIES

Researcher Dr. Friedrich F. Sander concluded that all severe illnesses, including **cardiac infarction** and **stroke**, are accompanied by a latent acidosis—i.e., hidden over-acidification, as in **diabetes mellitus, rheumatism, arthritis, and others**. Sander proved that latent acidosis in the tissues prepares the foundation for many illnesses *(The Acid-Base Household of Human Organism,* Hippokrates Publishing, 1985).

A study on 30 **obese women with increased blood-insulin** valence (University Bloemfontein in South Africa) has been published in the *American Journal of Clinical Nutrition* in 1994, No. 60, pages 48–53 (Slabber, M. et al.: Effects of low-insulin-response, energy-restricted diet on weight loss and plasma insulin concentrations in hyperinsulinemic obese females).

In a clinical scientific study on **diabetics** in 1980s, Dr. Ludwig Walb showed that after four to six weeks urine sugar measurements were reduced by 98% and the blood sugar measurements by 90%. The insulin-units could be reduced by 37%. The blood circulation improved. In five of his test subjects, the amputation of toes, foot, or lower leg could be avoided.

In a clinical scientific study in 1980, Dr. Ludwig Walb studied 620 patients from different disease groups. The serum **cholesterol** normalized within four weeks after changing to scientific eating in 86% of the cases.

In a clinical scientific study in 1978, Dr. Ludwig Walb studied 82 female and 51 male patients with an average of 58 years. The patients suffered from several illnesses, such as **disease of the heart and blood circulation** and the digestion organs, **diabetes, kidney diseases, rheum, tumors,** and **allergies**. The examined laboratory values improved by 80% in these four weeks. Particularly, the test was about following measurement sizes: white blood cells, calcium, Gamma GT, GPT and GOT, AP, erythrocyte sedimentation rate, uric acid, creatinin, urea nitrogen and urea, the proteins, as well as different blood fats, triglyceride, and entire cholesterol.

In a clinical scientific study in 1990, Dr. Walb proved that scientific eating reduces coagulation clotting (measured by the "quick-value").

Dr. Walb proved in the laboratory that the quick-value for coagulation was lowered by scientific eating for 80% of his test persons. The recovery had been so successful because the blood became less viscous, which in turn reduced the risk of **cardiac infarction, thrombosis, and stroke**. Test persons with **heart and circulatory** problems were urged to avoid denatured food but instead were told to eat several smaller portions during the day. These test persons reported immediate relief.

In a clinical scientific study in 1984, Dr. Walb proved that over 90% of patients with high blood **cholesterol** levels reduced those levels after only four weeks of scientific eating; the origin of **arteriosclerosis** and its consequences, the calcification of coronary artery vessels and the burden of the circulation of blood, was essentially reduced.

Dr. Kilmer McCully linked in his research **homocysteine** to vitamin B deficiency. His findings were published in 1997.

In a clinical scientific study on 120 test persons who suffered from incurable kidney disease, Dr. Walb proved that higher levels of fluid excretion provide relief for the **heart and kidneys;** 80% of those incurable patients recovered or at least improved.

The Russian Nobel Prize recipient Ivan Pavlov performed experiments on dogs. Minced (cooked) meat fed to the dogs, was digested within approximately four hours. (Carbohydrates required 1.5 hours, or less.) But when Pavlov fed cooked meat and carbohydrates together to the dogs, their digestion was delayed considerably. Instead of the approximately four hours that the dogs usually needed for digesting the cooked meat, it took eight hours or longer for this incompatible food to pass through their stomachs to the duodenum and small intestines.

Researcher Dr. Berthold Kern concluded that cardiac infarctions and strokes are "acid-catastrophes."

In a clinical scientific study, Dr. Seyle and a team of Swiss researchers concluded that arteriosclerosis, condensed and altered vascular side, will improve or even normalize by eating according to scientific eating.

Furthermore, he pointed out that all serious illnesses such as diabetes mellitus, rheumatism, and arthritis, are accompanied by a latent acidosis.

Researcher Dr. Krone of the Max Planck Institute in Germany proved that the metabolism of cells could be altered in a positive sense as well as a negative sense through food.

APPENDIX II

A Big Piece of the BioChemical Machine Puzzle
Some Background on Enzymes

Enzymes are biological catalysts capable of speeding up the chemical reactions necessary for life. However, regardless of what diet gurus say, enzymes do not possess magical properties that allow them to transcend the laws of body chemistry and "burn up calories before they hit your hips."[43]

In the last 30 years, as hundreds of enzymes have been identified in laboratory settings, it was believed that for every food there was an enzyme that would completely digest it, regardless of incompatible eating habits.

It's true that each chemical reaction in digestion requires its own particular enzyme. Digestive enzymes include amylase, which digests starch, lipase, which digests fats, and protease, which includes pepsin and is responsible for digesting proteins. Other enzymes play a part in the conversion of food energy into ATP (adenosine triphosphate), the power source for all cells in the body.

BUT, and here is the BIG BUT, for enzymes to reach their full effectiveness they require certain conditions, such as the right temperature, pH level, the availability of water, the right concentration, and the absence *of obstructive matter.* Temperature above 140°F/60°C damages (denatures) the intricate structure of enzymes, causing reactions to cease. Also, each enzyme operates best within a specific pH range and is denatured by *excessive acidity.* Acidity will prevent enzymes from speeding up the chemical reactions necessary for life. [44]

As you know, the A&B principles are all about avoiding excessive acidity, or the "obstructive matter" which reduces the effectiveness of enzymes.

The key to enzymes is to create an environment with a specific pH level that will allow them to operate effectively. By eating according to the A&B Method *the enzymes amylase and pepsin* will not be able *to hinder each other.*

Let's go back to our discussion of digestion, the switchboard of our very existence. According to *The World Book Encyclopedia:*

The digestive system consists primarily of the alimentary canal. As food moves through this canal, it is ground and mixed with various digestive juices. Most of these juices contain **digestive enzymes, chemicals that speed up reactions involved in the breakdown of food***. When digestion is completed, starches and complex sugars are broken down into simple sugars; fats are digested to fatty acids and glycerol, and proteins are digested to amino acids and peptides. Simple sugars, fatty acids, glycerol, amino acids and peptides are the digested foods that can be absorbed into the bloodstream. The digestive juice in the stomach is called gastric juice. It contains hydrochloric acid and the enzyme pepsin. This juice begins the digestion of protein foods-starches, sugars, and fats are not digested by the gastric juice.* [45]

Why can't starches like bread be digested by the same gastric juice your body employs to break down cooked meat, cooked eggs and homogenized/pasteurized milk? Because the stomach is too acidic—the enzyme amylase that is necessary to break down starches can't possibly work. It loses its effectiveness when mixed with pepsin.

What happens to carbohydrates (starches, sugars), since they are *not* digested by the same gastric juice that breaks down proteins? Remember, carbohydrate digestion is different from extremely-bad and bad protein digestion. A very important step in carbohydrate digestion occurs in the mouth. As you chew, the digestive enzyme amylase found in the saliva begins to split the starches and sugars into lower forms, preparing it for further reduction in the small intestine. Amylase acts best in an environment of positive alkalinity. Without an alkaline base there is no action of amylase on carbohydrate-rich foods. The slightest acid reaction slows down the splitting process and finally arrests this process of starchy reduction—*the food will not be completely digested.*

Also from *The World Book Encyclopedia:*

*In the small intestine, the digestive process is completed on the partially digested food by pancreatic juice, intestinal juice, and bile. The pancreatic juice is produced by the pancreas and pours into the small intestine through a tube, or duct. The pancreatic juice contains the enzymes trypsin, amylase, and lipase. Trypsin breaks down the partly digested proteins, amylase changes starch into simple sugars, and lipase splits fats into fatty acids and glycerol. **When the food is completely digested,** it is absorbed by tiny blood and lymph vessels in the walls of the small intestine. It is then carried by the bloodstream, throughout the body. Food particles are small enough to pass through the walls of the intestine and blood vessels—**but only when they are completely digested.**[45]*

If you don't eat according to your body chemistry by following the A&B Method, you will be unable to completely digest your food. None of the intestinal enzymes will function optimally in anything less than a positive alkaline medium. The alkaline state is maintained from the small intestine to the colon, or we could not digest our foods in the small intestine. If you eat incompatible mixtures of food, you create acidity that hinders the activity of your enzymes. Saliva, with its amylase, initiates starch digestion, *only* if the medium is alkaline, not otherwise. The gastric juice, with its pepsin, initiates protein digestion *only* if the medium is acid, not otherwise. The laws of your body chemistry are non-negotiable.

BioChemical Fact: Excessive acidity is the *corpus delicti* for most of our health and weight problems. When we eat in a chemically incompatible way, we hinder the enzymes from "speeding up" their chemical reactions, which slows down the metabolism. This, in turn, is the reason we get fat, fatigued, and ill.

Truth never dies. And the truth is that the enzyme amylase can't be optimally effective without an alkaline base and the enzyme pepsin can't be optimally effective if disturbed by amylase.

Enzymes work best in a specific pH range and are hindered or even denatured by excessive acidity and alkalinity. But your body will create no problem for you *when the food is completely digested.*

Acid-building (bad and extremely bad) protein digestion is different from Neutral protein and carbohydrate digestion.

If you ignore this fact then you are demanding too much from your buffer system. Plainly put, you have to make sure that your foods are completely digested, so that no acidity will denature your enzymes. In this case, perhaps even the diet guru I mentioned before would be able to live up to her promise that *you burn up calories before they hit your hips.*[43]

APPENDIX III

A Bit About Dr. Hay's Studies

Dr. William Howard Hay graduated from New York University on March 26, 1891, and practiced medicine and general surgery. After 16 years of practice devoted largely to general surgery, Dr. Hay came down with Bright's disease, an "incurable" kidney disease, accompanied by high blood pressure and a dilated heart. He received opiates and conventional treatment. Nothing helped, and he didn't recover. "There is no relief in medicine, but temporary relief," Dr. Hay said. It was this illness that changed Dr. Hay's view about medicine and surgery forever.

It was this key experience that led to his revolutionary discovery. He remembered an old report of a colonel in the British Army Medical Service, Robert McCarrison, who documented his observations and conclusions about the eating habits of the native people in India. Dr. Hay had nothing to lose. Immediately, he began eating like the native Himalayans.

Dr. Hay's medical problems slipped away. At the end of three months, he was again able to run long distances without distress. His weight dropped from 225 to 175 pounds. Years seemed to fall away, and he felt younger and stronger than he had in a long time. "It required a personal breakdown and a hopeless outlook for the future to really open [my] eyes to the possibilities of relief from disease along entirely different lines, however unorthodox these at first seemed," he said.

Based on his experiences and observations of the Himalayan's diet, Hays came to the conclusion that "all forms of disease and weight problems fall under one head—chemical imbalances of the body—and all are subject to restoration to the normal through correction of the body chemistry."

Dr. Hay closed his practice and founded his research institute in Pennsylvania where he dedicated 15 years to performing clinical research to develop and prove his theories about the acid-alkaline balance and the vital alkaline reserve. He started to publish his work which received a highly gratifying response. "The few thousands who have already benefited by resident treatment are but small in comparison to the thousands who have benefited through reading of the methods or studying and following the home course of management. The letters of thankfulness and appreciation received daily from so many who are complete strangers testify to the fact that the methods are so simple and effective that they can be successfully applied at any distance from personal supervision," he said.

NOTES

1. William Howard Hay: *A New Health Era,* Pocono Haven Publishing, 1933–1936.
2. IBID, page 140.
3. *NBC News,* January 6, 1997
4. Ragnar Berg: *Wholesome Food Nutrition for Mother and Child,* 5. Edition, Humata, 1986.
5. Friedrich F. Sander: *The Acid-Base Household of Human Organism,* Hippokrates, 1999.
6. Eduard Brecht: *Your Nutrition Is Your Destiny,* 6. Edition, Gewuerzmuehle, 1986.
7. Herman Aihara: *Basic Macrobiotics,* et al., Mahajiva Publishing, 1998.
8. B. Brenner: *Dietary Protein Intake and the Progressive Nature of Kidney Disease,* The New England Journal of Medicine 307, 632—No. 11, 1982.
9. Richard G. Klein: *The Human Career, Human Biological and Cultural Origins,* The University of Chicago Press, 1989.
10. Julian Jaynes: *The Origin of Consciousness in the Breakdown of the Bicameral Mind,* Houghton Mifflin, 1990.
11. American Diabetes Association.
12. CNN News, June 3, 1997.
13. Quazi S. Al Tariq, M.D., Horton Hospital (affiliate of New York Presbyterian Hospital), Arden Hill Hospital, Mid-Hudson Forensic Psych. Center, Goshen Residential Center.
14. IBID, Hay p. 42.
15. IBID, Tariq.
16. IBID, Tariq.
17. IBID, Tariq.
18. IBID, Tariq.
19. IBID, F.F. Sander.
20. IBID, Tariq.
21. CNN, *Headline News,* November 1996.
22. Hans Hermann Joergensen: *The Happy Molecule. Introduction into The Biochemistry of Minerals*; *with the Buffer-Capacity Raises and Falls Energy,* Medical Science, 6/93, 1988; *Acid-Alkaline Household—a Praxis-Near Procedure to Determine the Buffer-Capacity,* 5/2/1985, pp. 372–377 Medical Journal for Empirical Medical Science.
23. Eric Abraham Forsgren: *About the Rhythm of Liver-functions, Metabolism and Sleep,* Gumpert Publishing Gothenburg/Sweden.

24. Hilka de Groot-Boehlhoff, Professor Jutta Farhadi: *Issue of Nutrition,* Europe Textbook, 1989.
25. IBID, Groot-Boehlhoff, Farhadi.
26. American Heart Association, September 1998.
27. Claus Leitzmann, Professor of Nutrition, Justus Liebig University, Giessen.
28. American Dietetic Association, Publication: *A Primer on Fats and Oils.*
29. IBID, Groot-Boehlhoff, Farhadi.
30. Kilmar McCullym: *Homocysteine Revolution,* Group West, 1997.
31. *The Handy Science Answer Book,* p. 298, Visible Ink, 1994; Webster's New World Encyclopedia, p. 243; IBID, Groot-Boehlhoff, p. 63.
32. Judy Lin Eftekhar: *Feed Yourself Right,* Globe Communications, 1997, p. 43.
33. IBID, Groot-Boehlhoff, p. 128.
34. Professor Dr. Helmut Minne, M.D. (internal medicine) University Heidelberg; Chairman of the Board of Directors of the Kuratorium Knochengesundheit, e.v. (Kuratorium bone-health); Medical Director at Clinic The Fuerstenhof, Bad Pyrmont.
35. IBID, Eftekhar, p. 33.
36. *Webster's New World Encyclopedia,* p. 743.
37. *NBC Extra,* August 4, 1997.
37a. National Heart, Lung and Blood Institute
38. IBID, Groot-Boehlhoff.
39. IBID, Eftekhar, p. 11.
40. Osteoporosis Foundation, CNN, January 9, 1997.
41. IBID, Hay.
42. IBID, Hay.
43. Good Housekeeping, July 1996, p. 104
44. IBID, Groot-Boehlhoff, p. 230
45. Webster's New World Encyclopedia, pp. 202, 203.

BIBLIOGRAPHY

Aihara, Herman.
—*Basic Macrobiotics,* 1998.
—*Acid and Alkaline*, by Herman Aihara, Stan Hodson, 1986.
Milk, a Myth of Civilization, by Herman Aihara, Jacques De Langre Aihara, 1984.

Berg, Ragnar.
—*Wholesome Food Nutrition for Mother and Child,* Humata, 1986.
—*Dictionary of Foods*, Gaylord Hauser, Ragnar Berg, Benedict Lust Publications, 2002.

Brecht, Eduard. *Your Nutrition Is Your Destiny,* Gewuerz-muehle, 1986.

Brenner, B. *Dietary Protein Intake and the Progressive Nature of Kidney Disease,* New England Journal of Medicine 307, 632—No.11, 1982.

De Groot-Boehlhoff, Hilka, Professor Farhadi, Jutta.
—*The Issue of Nutrition,* Europe Textbook, Nourney, Vollmer Publishing, Europa NrL. 60312, 1989.

Forsgren, Eric Abraham, *About the Rhythm of Liver-Functions, Metabolism and Sleep,* Bocktruckerie Aktiebolag, Stockholm, Verlag I Marcus, 1935.

Jaynes, Julian. *The Origin of Consciousness in the Breakdown of the Bicameral Mind,* Houghton Mifflin, 1990.

Joergensen, Hans Hermann.
—*The Happy Molecule: Introduction into the Biochemistry of Minerals.*

—*With the Buffer Capacity Raises and Falls Energy,* Medical Science, 6/93/1988.
—*Acid-Alkaline Household—a Praxis-Near Procedure to Determine the Buffer Capacity,* Medical Journal for Empirical Medical Science.

Klein, Richard. *The Human Career, Human Biological and Cultural Origins,* The University of Chicago Press, 1989.

Leitzmann, Claus.
—*Dictionary of Nutrition/English/French/German/Italian/ Spanish,* Ulmer, 1996.
—Leitzmann, Claus, and Ibrahim Elmadfa: *Human Nutrition,* Ulmer 1999.
—Leitzmann, Claus, P. Glasauer, and J. Friedrich-Kaiser: *Food Aid in Form of Milkproducts,* Weltforum Publishing 1986.
—Leitzmann, Claus, Markus Keller, and Andreas Hahn: *Alternative Nutrition,* Hippokrates 1999.
—Leitzmann, Claus, Maria Weiger, and M. Kurz: *Nutrition [by] Cancer,* Graefe and Unzer 1996.

Ludwig, Walb.
—*Revolutionary Cognition in Health Management,* Medical Weekly 51,1940.
—*Rheumatic Problems of the Practitioner Once and Now,* Empirical Medical Science, 457, 1956
—*Prevention of Chemical Imbalances,* Medicine Today 1/8/1959.
—*Prophylaxis of Allergic Diseases,* Medicine Today 11/61.
—*Prophylaxis of Kidney Diseases,* Empirical Medical Science, 10/1962.
—*About the Influence of Meaningful Nutrition,* Empirical Medical Science, 9/13/1964.

—The Separation Cost, Especially for Kidney Diseases, Diaitia 6/1967.

—The Elektroneural-Diagnostic and—Therapy After Croon and the Significance of Objective Measured Data of Dysfunctional Body Functions. Physical Medicine and Rehabilitation, 7/9/1968.

—Simple Dietetics for the Practitioner. Magazine for General Medicine, 44, 29, 1968, 1434 ff.

—About the Effect of Separation Cost on Diabetes, Physical Medicine and Rehabilitation, 14, 9, 1973.

—Electro Diagnostic in the Practice, Empirical Medical Science, 4/24/1975.

—Dieting in Heart Therapy, Physical Medicine and Rehabilitation, 8/17/1976.

—Lecture About Croon's Method, Physical Medicine, 6/18/1977.

—Discussion Contribution to the Subject: Many Diet Concepts—Which One Should the Physician Follow in the Practice? Physical Medicine 8/18/1977.

—Detoxification with Separation Cost, Physical Medicine 6/21/1980.

—Nutrition Therapy with Separation Cost, Physical Medicine, 4/25/1984.

McCully, Kilmar. *Homocysteine Revolution,* Group West, 1997.

Sander, Friedrich. *The Acid-Base Household of Human Organism,* Hippokrates, 1999.

Seidl, Achim.
—The Emptiness of Zen, Diederichs Publishing, 1992.
—The Bi-Yaen-Lu, Hanser 1988.
—Psychosophie, Hanser 1992.

INDEX